FEARLESS BROTHS AND SOUPS

DITCH THE BOXES AND CANS WITH 60 SIMPLE RECIPES FOR REAL PEOPLE ON REAL BUDGETS

BY: CRAIG FEAR, NTP

www.FearlessEating.net

Published by Archangel Ink

ISBN: 1516962346
ISBN-13: 978-1516962341

Disclaimer

The information included in this book is for educational and informational purposes only and is not intended as a substitute for the medical advice of a licensed physician. I am not a medical doctor, and any advice I give is my opinion based on my own experience. As such, you should always seek the advice of your own health care professionals before acting upon anything I publish or recommend. By reading this book you agree that my company and I are not responsible for your health or the health of your dependents. Any statements or claims about the possible health benefits conferred by any foods have not been evaluated by the Food and Drug Administration and are therefore not intended to diagnose, treat, cure, or prevent any disease.

Table of Contents

Introduction

How to Reverse the #1 Nutritional Deficiency

Since I became a nutritional therapist back in 2008, I've met with hundreds of people with dozens of different health issues—weight issues, digestive issues, skin issues, autoimmune disorders, mental health issues, and so on. And I've also reached thousands more through my blog, Fearless Eating, my first book, *The 30 Day Heartburn Solution*, and my online digestive wellness e-course, Fearless Digestion.

Without question, I've identified the number one universal nutritional deficiency that unites the majority of all health problems. It's not minerals, vitamin D, omega-3s, or amino acids. And despite what all those bumper stickers say, you're not going to correct it by eating more kale.

The #1 nutritional deficiency is not something that can be confirmed by any epidemiological study or any scientific analysis.

But I can confirm it from my experience.

I call it . . .

Hypokitchenemia—a deficiency in knowledge for how to cook and prepare nutrient-dense foods in one's own kitchen.

Now, I know a lack of cooking skills is not technically a nutritional deficiency. But it will certainly lead to them.

The Challenge of Reversing Hypokitchenemia

We are more disconnected from where our food comes from than ever before in our history. Almost everything in conventional supermarkets comes from the realm of industrial agriculture, whose goal is not nourishment but rather cheap, nutrient-deficient food.

A bowl of Cheerios may be ready in ten seconds, Lunchables may be ready-made for your kids, and dinner may be ready in five minutes thanks to Campbell's and Progresso, but they're not anything your grandparents would have recognized as food.

And they're wreaking havoc on our health.

On the positive side, more and more people are becoming aware of the dangers of our food supply—GMOs, pesticides, animals raised in factory farms, high fructose corn syrup, trans fats, food colorings, preservatives, etc. The list goes on and on.

But the hard part is not waking up to the nightmares of industrial food. The hard part is avoiding it in a fast-paced culture that almost requires it.

And to avoid it, one must learn to cook. Of course, in today's world, when the demands on our time and money are viable concerns, we must learn to do it affordably and efficiently.

So therein lies the great challenge we all face in reversing hypokitchenemia.

Myself included.

However, there is one key thing we can all start doing to reverse this trend.

Reversing Hypokitchenemia with Fearless Broths and Soups

In my experience, one of the best ways to do this is to learn how to cook *REAL homemade* bone broths (also called bone stocks) and soups from scratch. *That* is what I mean by "fearless broths and soups." Clever take on my last name aside, it is truly a courageous step toward opting out of the industrial food system and reversing hypokitchenemia. And it's a great place to start for several reasons.

First, once you learn the basics for making broths, you'll be amazed at how quickly you can whip up some heart-stopping, fist-pumping, jaw-dropping, OMG THAT IS SO GOOD!-declaring, drop-dead-to-die-for-delicious soups.

Second, you can do it with real food sourced sustainably and cheaply. That's right, real homemade soups are one of the most *affordable* foods you can make when you're on a tight budget.

Third, they're one of the *healthiest* foods you can make. As you'll learn, homemade bone broths and soups supply your body with nutrients that support digestive health, bone health, joint health, insomnia and mental health, to name a few.

And finally, they're one of the *simplest* foods you can make, easily prepared in bulk so that you can have ready-made meals throughout the week.

Imagine for breakfast, instead of some nutrient-deficient boxed cereal that leaves you hungry an hour later, having a nourishing meal ready in just minutes that makes you feel sustained and alert all morning. This book will help you do that.

Imagine coming home from a busy day and having a healthy, satisfying dinner ready in five minutes. This book will help you do that.

Imagine being able to create a simple meal without the use of a recipe in just a few minutes. This book will help you do that.

Imagine reaching for broth in the morning instead of coffee and feeling calm and alert instead of jittery and neurotic.

"WHOAAAAAA, slow down there, dude! I am NOT giving up my morning coffee," you might be thinking. Admittedly, neither am I. But many people report they have, including many of my clients. So I'll just say that this book MAY help you do that.

If you think drinking broth in place of coffee is such a crazy idea, consider the New York City chef who opened a take-out window selling bone broths in to-go cups.

Regardless if you ever get to the point of trading your morning coffee for morning broth, this book will help you incorporate one of nature's most important foods in your diet on a regular basis without breaking the bank.

Best of all, one nourishing bowl of broth-based soup at a time, I'm confident you will slowly overcome hypokitchenemia and actually WANT to spend time in your kitchen.

Because if I can do it, ANYBODY can do it. You should know that I too once suffered with hypokitchenemia.

I grew up in the suburbs of Long Island during the 1980s, and for the first twenty years of my life, my great kitchen skill was toasting a bagel. Soup meant one of two things: Campbell's or Progresso. And broth certainly didn't come from bones. It came from a box, a can, or a bouillon cube.

It wasn't until I traveled to Burma, of all places, many years later, that a simple noodle soup would teach me some important lessons about the difference between the soup I grew up on and real soup from a real homemade bone broth. In the process, it helped me overcome hypokitchenemia and learn to LOVE making my own broths and soups.

My hope is that this book will do the same for you.

PART I:

THE LESSONS OF MOHINGA

Chapter 1

A Serious Addiction

Back in 2007, I traveled to Burma for two months. Now, Burma might not seem like the most popular destination on the globe, but the primary purpose of my trip was to deepen a Buddhist meditation practice I'd learned several years earlier. Burma is a deeply Buddhist country and, though not well traveled by many Westerners, offers many opportunities for the study and practice of meditation.

But meditation wasn't the only purpose of my trip. To be honest, I'm not the most noble of meditation practitioners. Too much meditation and I go a little stir-crazy. Being in a foreign place, naturally I wanted to experience the country outside the confines of meditation centers.

Little did I know that the secondary intention of my trip, to travel and see the country, would lead to a serious addiction.

The first time I tried it in Yangon (formerly called Rangoon), I knew I was hooked. From that point forward, I could not start my day without it, and I would do whatever it took to find the best sources.

On a few occasions, that meant wandering down a dark alley where few foreign travelers ever set foot and no English was spoken. The locals always knew why I'd come. Knowing head nods and sly smiles were the only form of communication needed.

But more commonly, to get my daily fix, it simply meant stepping right outside my hotel and getting it on the street.

Be it the cities of Yangon or Mandalay, small towns and villages, the sacred temples of Bagan, or even inside the meditation centers themselves, the source of my addiction was everywhere.

Mohinga.

Mohinga is the national dish of Burma, a traditional soup with such exquisite flavors that it's as if all the quintessential flavors of Southeast Asia come together in perfect balance and harmony. Though technically not a drug, in the Buddhist sense (where everything within the net of our senses can cause intense craving and desire), it's pretty damn close.

Mohinga starts with a fish broth. Now that may not sound very exciting, but it's what's added to that broth that makes it so divinely delicious. Lemongrass, banana stem, ginger, garlic, and onions slowly simmer away and infuse the broth with both an herbal, lemony sweetness and a pungent earthiness. Fish sauce gives the broth a subtle-but-not-too-subtle fish essence, and fresh local fish gives it all a hearty boost.

But that's only the beginning.

All of that sweet, sour, salty deliciousness is then ladled over rice noodles and served with sides of fresh lime, dried red chilies, cilantro, and more fish sauce. You add as much or as little as you want, depending on your personal tastes. Hard-boiled eggs, crispy fried onions, a crispy fish cake, and other herbs and spices are often part of the broth and accompaniments as well. Different areas of the country have different interpretations and ingredients. Yangon mohinga is slightly different that Mandalay mohinga and so forth.

And in Burma, they primarily have it for breakfast. I would wake up with such a craving for it that I could barely function until I had my fill. It is hands down the greatest soup I've ever had, and if I ever go back to Burma, my primary purpose will be for mohinga.

Spiritual enlightenment is now a distant second.

The purpose of this little travelogue is not to show off my exotic travel experiences but rather to highlight five specific things that mohinga can teach us about real broths and soups.

Chapter 2

Lesson #1 - Every Country Has Its Mohinga

If you were to travel around the world, especially in Asia, you'd find mohinga in different disguises almost everywhere. Steaming cauldrons of soup are an everyday part of street fare, street markets, and tiny little cafes with makeshift kitchens, often in full view, adjacent to the seating area.

Just like mohinga in Burma, every country has its staple soups with an almost infinite amount of simple variations. There are thousands of noodle soups, rice soups, and soups with legumes, grains, different meats, seafood, vegetables, spices, and herbs.

Some of these soups have become familiar to us in melting-pot America. Vietnamese pho, Thai tom yum, Japanese miso soup, Indian mulligatawny, and Chinese egg drop soup are just a few names you might recognize.

Despite the bewildering variety, there is one universal feature that unites all traditional soups across the globe. They all start with a ***properly prepared*** bone broth (which you'll learn to make in Part II). Basically, all that means is animal bones that have been simmered in water for extended periods of time.

This simmering does three things in particular. First, it leaches out nutrients and presents them in highly absorbable form to our bodies. Second, it helps to develop flavor. Vegetables like onions, carrots, and celery are often added for additional nutrients and flavor. And third, it creates a simple, inexpensive base for a diverse range of soups and stews such as bisques, chowders, porridges, congees, bouillabaisses, cioppinos, gumbos, borschts, tagines, and curries.

To drive home the point, in the 1930s, Dr. Weston Price, a dentist from America, traveled the earth and studied the diets of traditional cultures untouched by civilization. Whether in Alaska, Africa, Europe, Australia, or Asia, Dr. Price made the connection between the people's excellent health and their native diets. And their native diets ALWAYS included bone broths.

But you don't have to travel to the opposite ends of the earth to experience these wonderful dishes as the United States has its own traditions. Our grandparents and great-grandparents brought the Old World recipes with them, recipes that were passed down for hundreds, if not thousands, of years.

If you're old enough, you surely have fond memories of the wonderful scents that would permeate the kitchen from steaming pots of broth and soup. Prior to World War II, a stockpot was a part of every kitchen, simmering slowly, sometimes for days at a time. And you surely remember the mouthwatering classic recipes that were staples in your family.

If you're Italian, you might remember wedding soup, pasta e fagioli (pasta and beans), minestrone, or stracciatella (a type of egg drop soup). If you're French, maybe it's French onion soup, bouillabaisse, vichyssoise, or some sort of seafood bisque. If you're from eastern Europe, it could be borscht, goulash, vegetable and barley, or split pea soup. If you're Asian, it's some sort of hot and sour, curry, noodle, or coconut milk-based soup.

Whatever your ethnicity, your ancestors took their traditions with them to America and maintained them for a few generations until at least the early to mid-twentieth century. After World War II, supermarkets, fast food, and industrial agriculture eroded our cooking traditions, and our food system basically went to hell. And a very sad, but somewhat funny thing, has happened since then. I've been confronted with this over and over again when I meet with clients. Let's head back to Asia one last time to understand this more fully.

Chapter 3

Lesson #2 - Mohinga Comes From REAL Markets, NOT Supermarkets

Besides devouring multiple bowls of mohinga in one sitting, my next favorite thing about Asia was visiting the markets that supplied the raw ingredients for the traditionally prepared broths and soups. It was and still remains the thing I most adored about the places I visited.

Let's just say the markets of Asia are a liiiiittle different than the supermarkets of America. For someone like me who grew up going to supermarkets, the markets of Asia provide quite a shocking contrast. Nothing comes in boxes and cans. There are no confusing nutrition labels, no soul-numbing elevator music, no depressing fluorescent lighting, and no disgruntled minimum-wage workers. Everything is fresh, everything is local, and everything feels ALIVE.

Asian markets are often outdoors, operate rain or shine, and take over entire city streets, village streets, sidewalks, alleyways, and parks. The vivid colors, the succulent smells of herbs and spices, curries and simmering soups, the bizarre and exotic fruits and vegetables, the busy flow of people and animals, carts and mopeds, intersecting, weaving, and flowing together sweeps you into an almost trance-like state of sensory stimulation.

But besides all the vibrant life, there's also a lot of death. And it's right in front of you. And it can be really shocking. And this is certainly a huge difference compared to American supermarkets.

Fresh-caught seafood—fish, shrimp, eels, shellfish, crabs, and squid—is often still squirming and crawling in their buckets. Pigs' heads, pigs' feet, whole chickens with the heads still on, chicken parts (like feet and gizzards), lamb and cow parts (including different bones, large cuts of meat, ribs, and tails) are all on display too. People tell me of similar experiences in the markets of other areas of the world—Europe, South America, Africa, etc.

This is significant for our purposes because a truly nutrient-rich broth often contains more than just bones but also additional animal parts such as joints, tendons, backs, tails, necks, and heads. You'll see in the next lesson that these parts contain valuable nutrients that are hard to obtain in other foods. Of course, using these parts tends to horrify so many of us in America, especially those of us raised in cities and suburbs. But the reality of death is the same in American supermarkets as it is in Asian markets. It's just kept hidden from us.

Rarely will you see bones for sale anymore, which are an essential component of making a good broth. So many of our meats our deboned, trimmed of fat, and packaged as boneless breasts and filets. And rarely do you see the parts of animals that are highly valued and on display in Asian markets—feet, necks, heads, tails, etc. In fact, many of those parts are shipped off to Asia from American processing plants! And something quite bizarre has happened as a result.

Millions of Americans have become afraid of real food.

I see this over and over when I work with clients. Because bone broths are so beneficial for many health issues, especially digestive problems, I ask most of my clients to start making bone broths at home. The objections I receive are often shocking and, well, sometimes funny. Sometimes I have to bite my lip when one of my adult clients makes a squirmy face like a little child at the sheer mention of making a broth with actual bones.

"Wait, are you saying you want me to use actual BONES?!"

"Chicken feet? Are you SERIOUS?!"

"Ew. Gross."

That's just a small sample of the common reactions I get. People say kids are picky eaters but in my experience, adults can be a lot worse.

And bone broths are just the tip of the iceberg. Jessica Prentice in her wonderful cookbook, *Full Moon Feast*, writes:

> *"All too often, modern Americans are like oversized infants when it comes to food. We are used to having it provided for us. We are like baby birds in a nest with our mouths wide open, squawking for more. But we never grow up into the mama bird that goes and hunts and finds food and provides. We never learn how to feed ourselves, because it is so easy and culturally supported not to. People who cook on a daily basis and who like to prepare food from scratch are considered either foodies or health nuts. Cooking is not seen as a universal skill of self-sufficiency and adulthood, like driving a car. We are surprised when someone doesn't know how to drive a car, but we are not at all surprised when someone doesn't know how to cook. Large corporations are more than happy to keep us in this state of helplessness. It creates a huge market for factory-processed products and fast food."*[1]

And it also keeps us afraid of food because we no longer process it ourselves. It wasn't too long ago when you wouldn't see this fear of food in America. Before the rise of Campbell's, Progresso, and store-bought broths, we made broths ourselves. We butchered our own animals, used all parts of the animals, and worked in tight-knit communities to raise food together. I love listening to older folks speak with warmth and fondness for the freshly prepared foods of their parents and grandparents. I often

---

[1] Jessica Prentice, *Full Moon Feast* (White River Junction, VT: Chelsea Green Publishing, 2006), 247–248.

hear a tinge of sadness in their voices as they recall these foods not just for their taste but for their connection to a simpler time.

Of course, our food system has changed dramatically in the past fifty years or so. Now we let the food industry raise and process our animals for us. Worse, the animal products in most mega-supermarkets come from factory farms where they are kept in confined spaces and fed unnatural food and growth hormones that fatten them faster than a natural, free-range, pastured environment. Not surprisingly, they get sick in these unnatural conditions and are given tons of antibiotics. This is a good reason to start sourcing your food from real farms and real farmers who treat their animals humanely. And that is a truly fearless act in today's world where convenience and cost usually trump conscience and awareness. Waking up to the horrors of our food system takes commitment. It also takes a little courage sometimes.

But don't worry. I'm not going to make you start butchering your own animals. Nor do any of the bone broth recipes here absolutely require the use of animal parts like feet and heads. Though recommended, they're always optional. But you will need to start using bones.

Seeing as how you have this book in your hands (or on your computer screen), I'm going to assume that using bones isn't too much of an objection for you. But if it does freak you out, I promise you'll get over it quickly, because when you start to make properly prepared broths on a regular basis, slowly simmered from real bones, you will be amazed at the incredibly delicious soups you will make from them. Store-bought soups can NEVER compare to the real thing.

Doing it in a way that saves you time and money will help too. And if you have a chronic health issue, as most of us do today, you'll probably start feeling better, too. For most people, that's the real game changer. All previous fears of food evaporate in the presence of improved digestion, better sleep, more energy, and clearer thinking. Contrary to popular belief, there's incredible life-giving, healing properties in all those bones and unwanted parts. Just ask your grandma! She may not have been a scientist, but she's observed over and over how a chicken soup helps one recover from the common cold, indigestion, and all types of health issues.

I can attest to all the clients I've worked with that are amazed at the healing power of broths and soups. When heartburn, IBS, chronic bloating, chronic joint pain, intense sugar cravings, and insomnia all start resolving, there's very little hesitation to use bones and animal parts anymore. Many start seeking out good sources in their communities and even become OK with those animal parts that previously grossed them out. So let's understand why real homemade broths and soups are so beneficial to our health.

Chapter 4

Lesson #3 - Mohinga Keeps Us Glued Together

Much has been said about the health benefits of bone broths in recent years. Many bloggers, podcasts, and authors are helping us understand, on a scientific level, why the stockpot was such an essential part of our grandparents' kitchens. Scientific analysis of properly made broth reveals dozens of highfalutin, hard-to-pronounce nutrients like proteoglycans, glycosaminoglycans, hyalauronic acid, and chondroitin sulfates.

But for our purposes, I want to focus on just one for now, collagen, which at the very least is easy to pronounce.

Collagen comes from the Greek word "kolla," which literally means glue, and it's the substance that in many ways keeps us glued together. It's made up of proteins that form the strong but pliable connective tissues in animals (including us) that stretch, bend, and jiggle—notably, tendons, ligaments, cartilage, joints, and skin.

An overly simplistic but perhaps useful analogy might be to think of collagenous tissues like a rubber band as it provides a better visual for what can happen as we age. Over time, rubber bands lose their elasticity and become brittle and weak. This is kind of like what happens to the collagen in our body as we get older. Tendons and ligaments lose their flexibility, skin sags, and joints lose their suppleness. However, we can slow this process down by giving our bodies the raw materials to keep us jiggling and moving well into old age. One of the best sources is, of course, bone broths. That's why a good bone broth will contain more than just bones but also those collagen-rich animal parts like heads, tails, and feet that tend to freak people out.

For a chicken broth, that could mean the backs, necks, and/or feet. For a beef broth, it could mean the oxtail or a calf's foot. And for a good fish broth, as in the case of mohinga, it would include some fish heads.

You can actually see proof of a collagen-rich broth when it cools. It will literally gel and jiggle like Jell-O. This is a good thing! That gelling comes from gelatin, which is simply collagen that has been broken down during the simmering process.

Gelatin has many health benefits, but in particular, it has been prized for centuries around the world for its ability to help ease gastrointestinal problems. Dr. Kaayla Daniel, in her thoroughly researched article, entitled "Why Broth is Beautiful," discusses the role gelatin played in the medical profession in the first part of the twentieth century. She cites numerous researchers who studied its benefits and doctors who used it therapeutically with patients for an assortment of digestive problems, including bacterial infections, inflammation, heartburn, IBS, and dysbiosis. In particular, she focuses on the roles of proline and glycine, the two main amino acids in gelatin, which have a multitude of healing and protective effects.[2]

Gelatin also contains glutamine, another amino acid, which helps fuel and regenerate the mucosal lining of the small intestine. This can help with celiac disease and inflammatory conditions like colitis, ulcers, and Crohn's disease.

Gelatin has hydrophilic properties, too, meaning it attracts water. Thus, it acts as sort of a lubricant and can help facilitate

---

[2] Dr. Kaayla Daniel, "Why Broth Is Beautiful: Essential Roles for Proline, Glycine and Gelatin," *Weston A. Price Foundation,* June 18, 2003, http://www.westonaprice.org/health-topics/why-broth-is-beautiful-essential-roles-for-proline-glycine-and-gelatin/.

food through the digestive system. This can help a wide variety of digestive issues, but especially chronic bloating and IBS.

And yet, it never ceases to amaze me just how much money people will spend on supplementation and then complain about the cost of real food.

Why Bone Broths Are Better Than Supplements

You can certainly pay hundreds of dollars for digestive supplements like glutamine, deglycyrrhizinated licorice (DGL), aloe vera juice, and digestive enzymes, and those things certainly could help. But you could also experience the same gut-healing benefits by making homemade bone broth on a regular basis. And pay almost nothing.

Let's take a look at a few more common health conditions and see how bone broth can benefit.

Joint problems?

You can certainly pay over $40 for a bottle of glucosamine and/or chondroitin sulfates.

Glucosamine and chondroitin sulfates are types of large, gelatinous molecules called proteoglycans which help repair, lubricate, and cushion our joints. But you could also get those things in homemade bone broth and again, pay almost nothing.

Skin issues?

You can use all sorts of pricey prescription creams and even herbal beauty products, which may help. A common component you'll see in these products is hyalauronic acid, another proteoglycan that supports skin health. But it's naturally present in a properly made broth.

Insomnia?

Melatonin is a common over-the-counter remedy for poor sleep. But try consuming a homemade broth-based soup for dinner instead and see what happens. The glycine from gelatin also helps the body produce melatonin naturally.

Of course, broth also contains minerals that help to relax our muscles and contribute to bone broth's calming effect.

Personally, I never sleep better than when I have a good broth-based meal at dinner. And speaking of minerals...

Osteoporosis?

Many people think osteoporosis, a condition where bones become weak and brittle, is merely a calcium deficiency disease and therefore, regularly take calcium supplementation. If only it were that simple. There's *a lot more* to the integrity of bones than just calcium.

Bone is also made of other minerals like magnesium, potassium, and trace minerals, which a good bone broth will also contain. However, you need a lot more than just minerals to build and maintain healthy bones.

Bone contains only about 50 percent minerals, most of which makes up its hard outer layer, which gives bone its solid appearance. But bone is a *living tissue*. Inside is a complex matrix of metabolically active connective tissue composed of things like cartilage, nerves, blood cells, marrow, and collagen. Yes, collagen! Collagen keeps bones strong and pliable just as it does other tissues in our body. Think of your bones like a brick wall. The minerals act as the bricks themselves, and the collagen is the mortar between the bricks that glues and solidifies them together.

I could carry on with additional benefits of broths, but I think you get the point that broth keeps us well supported, well cushioned, and well lubricated, especially as we age. While aging is inevitable, chronic pain is not! Osteoporosis, knee and hip replacements, and the use of anti-inflammatory drugs for joint pain have become so widespread that most people just consider it "normal." And yet, we are sometimes amazed when we meet an older person who maintains a natural suppleness in their skin and a spring in their step. Chances are they are one of the very few who have maintained the traditional diets from their youth, which, of course, includes bone broths.

Chapter 5

Lesson #4 - The Natural Flavors of Mohinga Come from Actual Natural Flavors

This is another reason it's so important to start making your own homemade broths.

Store-bought broths and soups that come in cans and boxes lack not only the nutrient density of properly prepared homemade ones, but they also lack REAL flavor. To compensate, almost all store-bought broths, including organic ones, use added flavorings.

The worst brands use monosodium glutamate (MSG) and other chemical flavorings. And that includes the ubiquitous "natural flavors," which you'll see on the ingredient labels of tons of processed foods. Keep in mind that these "natural flavors" are created in labs, not nature. According to the FDA, if they are derived from previously naturally occurring substances, they can be legally termed "natural."[3] By law, food companies can use the term "natural flavors" to disguise a whole host of chemicals and to keep their secrets hidden from their competitors. Ain't the food industry just swell?

---

[3] "CFR - Code of Federal Regulations Title 21." *U.S. Food and Drug Administration,* last revised April 1, 2014, www.accessdata.fda.gov/scripts/cdrh/cfdocs/cfcfr/cfrsearch.cfm?fr=501.22.

"Natural flavors" allows food manufacturers to re-create, via chemical processes, the same flavor over and over and thus, the same product over and over. And that's good for business, but that's not how things work in nature. It's why if you were to go to Burma, you'd never have the same bowl of mohinga. Ever. Regional differences in plant and animal life, which change with the seasons, create regional differences in taste. Furthermore, subtle differences in herbs, spices, a little more of this, a little less of this, all contribute to wonderful variations in **actual natural flavors**! Of course, the same could be said for almost any real, natural food.

Bottom line, the purpose of "natural flavors" is flavoring, not nutrition.

And unfortunately, the organic ones aren't much better. They also rely heavily on flavorings. The more common ones you'll see are "natural chicken flavor" in organic chicken broth and "natural beef flavor" in organic beef broth. Again, they're not natural at all. Food companies can use those terms in the same way they use the term "natural flavors."

Another common one you'll see is "yeast extract." Yeast extract is derived from an industrial process that removes the cell walls of yeast to extract the contents. Mmmmmm, yeast extract. Doesn't that sound yummy? Just like Grandma used to make!

Well, truth be told, yeast extract actually does taste good. That's why it's in so many processed foods. Similar to MSG, it has a meaty taste. In fact, yeast extract contains the free glutamic acids in MSG that many people claim can cause adverse reactions in the nervous system and brain. It's very controversial whether or not these free glutamic acids (which occur naturally in nature) are concentrated enough in the flavorings of processed foods to cause harm to the body, but what's absolutely not controversial is that **yeast extract is a flavor enhancer**.

Let's understand how real homemade broths develop actual natural flavors and why store-bought versions can never duplicate the real thing. I've come up with a simple formula to explain it.

Time + Quality + Variety = Flavor

Let's look at each one separately.

Time

Real bone broths need *time* to develop flavor. As bones simmer in water over time, nutrients leach out, which contribute to their flavor. Meaty bones in particular will help to develop flavor. Additions of real herbs, real spices, and real vegetables like carrots, onions, and celery will also add more flavor.

Of course, time is the enemy of processed foods. The more time things take to produce, the less profitable they are. I don't know exactly how long store-bought broths are simmered. They don't tell you. But it certainly can't be very long, otherwise they wouldn't have to use flavorings! And you'll often see things like "onion powder" or "carrot puree" or "celery juice concentrate" instead of actual herbs and vegetables, which, of course, cost companies more.

Quality

Second, a good broth will contain *good-quality* bones. The better the diet and treatment of animals, the healthier they are and the more nutrients that leach out of their bones.

Conventional store-bought broth from companies like Campbell's, College Inn, Swanson, and Kitchen Basics are certainly using factory farm-raised animal bones. Organic companies like Full Circle, Imagine, and Nature's Promise may source better quality bones, but it's unlikely they're using a variety.

Variety

And finally, as we've seen, a good bone broth uses not just bones but a *variety* of other collagen-rich animal parts that impart valuable nutrients such as gelatin! Store-bought broth is NEVER gelatinous, organic or not.

Chapter 6

Lesson #5 - There is No Authentic Recipe for Mohinga in This Book

Truth be told, mohinga is somewhat complicated to make. And the purpose of this book is not to make your life more complicated. However, there is a *simplified* recipe for mohinga in this book! And that's because all the recipes included will emphasize simplicity. They're geared to all you stressed out moms and dads, workaholics, and hypokitchenemics trying to figure out how to eat well with limited funds and time. And these days, that's just about everyone.

Now I'm not trying to sugar coat things, either. There will be some investment of time up front when making the broths, but it's incredibly simple. And once you make the broth, you'll have a base for whipping up any meal of the day in a matter of minutes.

Here are five more reasons making broths and soups at home will save you time and money:

1. You can make them in bulk.

It takes just as much time to make a quart of broth as it does to make twenty quarts. And it takes just as much time to make a bowl of soup as it does eight bowls of soup. Making large batches doesn't cost much more either.

2. They can be reheated faster than most microwaveable meals.

Make a large pot of soup at the beginning of the week. For quick meals the rest of the week, all you have to do is warm up a bowl. They're cheaper than most microwaveable meals, too— and needless to say, healthier.

3. You can have broth for breakfast!

So many people complain that they don't have time for breakfast. Warming up a bowl of broth with some veggies, some eggs, and some spices barely takes any time at all. And it'll cost you less than an Egg McMuffin. In fact, I have an entire chapter dedicated to this!

4. Bones are cheap!

Farmers, fishmongers, butchers, and even supermarkets will give them to you at incredibly reasonable prices, if not free, because so few people value them anymore. And of course, you can save and stockpile bones in your freezer from different types of meat. More on all this in Chapter 8.

5. They don't require advanced cooking skills.

Place bones in a pot of water. Simmer them. Bam. You're a broth-making expert. No $50,000 culinary degree required.

Of course, there's a little more to it than that, but not that much. So now that you know WHY making homemade broths is so important, let's finally get into the nitty-gritty of making them.

PART II

FEARLESS BONE BROTH BASICS

Chapter 7

Two Big Ideas for Making Broths

There are two important ideas to keep in mind before we get started:

1. Be a cook, not a chef.

First, this book is NOT about the finer techniques of making broths and soups. I'm not a chef, and I'm not interested in making you a chef. I'm interested in making you a cook.

Big difference.

Chefs know how to control the process of making broths for different textures, subtle flavors, and appearances. That's fine when preparing them for paying customers and food critics.

I'm more interested in getting you comfortable with the basics so that you can bring them into your life on a consistent basis. For that reason, there are no techniques in here for making things like consommés or double-cooked broths. As I've learned with my clients, the more complicated I make things, the less likely they'll succeed.

Which leads me to the second big idea and, in my opinion, the most important tip I can share:

2. When you simmer bones in water, good things happen.

Burn that big idea into your memory and always refer to it when you're not exactly sure what you're doing is correct.

So many people get their panties all up in a bunch (especially men) if you don't do it this way or that way.

You say bone stock, I say bone broth. For the most part, the words "stock" and "broth" are used interchangeably. Some say a bone broth is cooked for less time than a bone stock, and some say the complete opposite. Who cares? Probably chefs. See Big Idea #1.

Other differences in opinion include how long to simmer broths for, whether or not to roast bones first, and techniques for creating a gelatin-rich broth.

Listen, I don't care if you can only simmer your broth for one hour, if that's all the time you have. I don't care if it doesn't form gelatin. I don't care if you don't roast the bones first. I don't care if all you have are a few chicken bones. And I certainly don't care if you call it a stock or a broth. Call it a "witches' brew" if you want. Just put what you got in a pot, simmer it for as long as you can . . . and good things happen.

It will be infinitely better than anything you can buy in a store.

Chapter 8

Basic Broth Ingredients

Quality Bones and Animal Parts

Try to get the best quality bones and animal parts that you can. For fish, that means wild-caught fish. For chicken, that means chickens that are free to roam on pasture and eat their natural diet. For beef, that means pastured, grass-fed beef. You don't have to be obsessive about it, though. Do the best you can. I know it's not possible for everyone to get the best quality. Any bones you use will still be better than purchasing store-bought broths. Just know that conventionally raised animal parts will not be as nutrient-rich.

Finding Bones

Many people ask where they can find good-quality bones. Contact your local farmers first, in particular, your local farmers who are raising their animals on pasture. As already discussed, so few people value bones anymore that they'll probably be thrilled to give them to you at a very reasonable price, if not completely free. Next, try your local butcher or the meat department at your local health food store. They should have a steady supply and will often give them to you at a very reasonable price as well. You may also find a good supply from Asian supermarkets, if you have one near where you live. Other ethnic/international markets may be good sources as well. They're not always the best quality in these places, though, so be sure to ask whether or not the animals were raised on pasture.

Once you find a good source, try to get as many different types of bones and parts of the animal as possible. For example, for chicken stock, get some chicken necks, backs, and chicken feet. For beef stock, try to get an oxtail and use a combination of meaty bones, knuckle bones, and marrow bones. Some of these additional parts are easier to get than others, so if you can't get a good variety, it's no big deal. And if using chicken feet grosses you out, just skip it!

Save Your Bones!

Never throw bones out ever again! Build up your supply at home by saving bones in your freezer until you have enough to make a broth. It doesn't matter if they're cooked or raw. Both are equally good to use. And it's perfectly acceptable to combine bones from different animals. I'll often throw pork, chicken, and beef bones together.

Vegetables

Most broths also include a variety of vegetables. Vegetables impart additional nutrients and flavor. The classic vegetable combination is called a "mirepoix" and contains carrots, celery, and onions. But other vegetables are fine to add as well—garlic, leeks, scallions, shallots, turnips, mushrooms, peppers, and asparagus are common additions. Starchy root vegetables (which are fine to add in soups) and cruciferous vegetables (such as broccoli, Brussels sprouts, cauliflower and cabbage, which can be a little too bitter) are the only ones you want to avoid.

Save the scraps from all your vegetables—ends of onions, tips of carrots, stalks—put them in a freezer bag, and add them to your broth.

But don't worry if you don't have all the vegetables. Don't have celery? Don't worry about it. Forgot to get carrots? Skip 'em. Don't want to use any vegetables? No problem. In fact, some people feel the use of vegetables gives too strong of a flavor to broths. The great thing about broths is that you can easily spice them up even if they come out a little bland. Some prefer blander broths for that very reason. This is all a matter of personal preference. Experiment!

Herbs

The classic herb combination almost always includes thyme and some bay leaves. Other common herbs are rosemary, basil, parsley, and tarragon. Whole peppercorns are also a common addition.

Herbs impart nutrients but are mostly used for flavor. Referred to as a "bouquet garni," they are often tied together with some string and then removed when the broth is finished. In keeping with my pattern of annoying trained chefs everywhere, I usually throw them in untied and leave them in because I'm lazy. Also, I don't mind peppercorns and thyme twigs floating around in my soups. I just pick 'em out as I go (or in the case of peppercorns, eat them). Oftentimes, I won't use any herbs. They're not essential if you're not a chef. Are you seeing that I'm not a perfectionist about this stuff? (You needn't be one, either.)

Chapter 9

Basic Broth Kitchen Tools

For all the tools below, I've created a resources page on my website where you can find my recommended choices: http://FearlessEating.net/fearless-broths-and-soups-resources

Stockpot

There's very little you need except a good stockpot. If you're just starting out, a small, standard eight-quart stockpot is more than adequate. Keep in mind, though, by the time you add in the bones and other ingredients, you won't get much more than about four quarts of broth. Now four quarts might seem like a decent amount, but in time, I'm confident the soup recipes here will so nourish you and so excite your taste buds that you'll start going through broth faster than a chef in a busy restaurant. Don't be surprised if your family starts demanding them more often, too. I've had more than a few clients tell me how pleasantly surprised they were when their picky-eating kids started enjoying them. And if you start sharing your broths and soups with friends, expect more dinner and potluck invitations. So just be prepared that in time you'll probably want to make more than four quarts.

When you're ready, I'd highly recommend investing in a larger stockpot. I often use a twenty-quart stockpot from which I get about twelve quarts of broth, two-thirds of which I'll freeze. I also have eight- and twelve-quart stockpots to use when needed as well.

When choosing a good quality stockpot, make sure to pick one with a heavy-duty bottom. Stainless steel is always a good choice as well as stockpots with a protective enamel coating. Le Creuset, All-Clad, and Cuisinart are some companies that produce good-quality stockpots.

Crock-Pot

A Crock-Pot (also called a slow cooker) is perfectly fine to use in place of a stockpot, though you won't find many larger than about eight quarts. There's no question that Crock-Pots are a good option for those with concerns about leaving their stovetop on for long periods. However, one thing to consider is that Crock-Pots usually only have three settings—high, low, and warm. As you'll see in the next chapter, to create a gelatinous broth, you want to keep the broth at a *very gentle* simmer. Most Crock-Pots don't allow this. Usually both the high and low settings will boil liquids, while the warm setting keeps it just below a simmer. That being said, I've had many people report to me that despite this, their broth gelled beautifully. Creating gelatinous broths can sometimes be a hit or miss for other reasons as well. Chapter 13 will explain more about conditions that help to create gelatin-rich broths.

Pressure Cooker

Using a pressure cooker has become a trendy thing among bone broth enthusiasts lately. Pressure cookers dramatically reduce the time bone broths need to cook and supposedly still retain the nutrient value. From what I've researched, it seems like a viable and certainly ultra-quick way to make broth. The one big negative is that, again, you can't make more than a few quarts at once. I haven't used one, but you could certainly give it a try.

Fine Mesh Strainer

You can use any old strainer and line it with a piece of fine mesh cheesecloth or just use a fine mesh strainer. If you're straining a large amount of broth, it's helpful to have a larger, sturdier strainer, preferably with some handles that can rest over the sides of whatever pot you're straining the broth into.

Storage Containers

I recommend using wide-mouth glass mason jars for storage containers, but you could use any size or type of glass jars you want. I mostly use quart-sized ones but will often use half-gallon ones when making larger batches. I don't recommend plastic containers, but I will use them sometimes when I run out of glass jars. If using plastic, be sure the broth is thoroughly cooled before filling.

Chest Freezer

In time, the one larger purchase you may want to consider is a chest freezer or another type of small freezer. Trust me, once you get hooked on broths and soups, your kitchen freezer will fill up really fast. I now have a small chest freezer JUST for storing bones and broths.

Chapter 10

A Simple Five-Step Formula for Making Broths

The following formula is a good starting point for making almost any type of broth. It's also easily memorized because each step begins with the letter S. In a short time, you won't even need to follow a recipe to make a broth. Just follow this formula and you're good to go.

1. Soak

Soaking bones in water with a little vinegar helps to pull the minerals from the bones. Soak about 1–2 pounds of bones per quart of water. I never measure this, though. My gauge is filling whatever pot I'm using about half full with bones and then adding water to cover the bones. That's usually about right. For a standard eight-quart stockpot, add about 2–4 Tbsp vinegar if using chicken and about a ¼–½ cup if using beef bones. Let it sit for about 30–60 minutes. Note: Fish broth is the only broth where this step is often skipped.

2. Skim

After soaking, turn the heat up to high. Before it boils, some foam will start to form on the surface, which is called "scum." True to its name, it's not very pleasant looking, but it can't hurt you. Simply skim it off with a ladle or a small mesh strainer, which will easily latch onto the scum. You probably won't be able to skim off every last bit of it, but get as much as you can. Without skimming, the broth will become cloudier and the flavor will be slightly affected, but it's not that big of a deal. Different types of bones will produce more scum than others. Once you've skimmed the broth, add in your chopped vegetables. You could add them when soaking the bones too, but they'll float to the surface, and this can make skimming the scum more difficult.

3. Simmer

This is probably the most important step! The key is to GENTLY SIMMER and not boil the bones, which can damage the gelatin (but won't ruin the broth). So once the water has come to a boil and the scum forms, immediately turn down the heat. Simmering should only be slightly perceptible—a few bubbles rising to the surface here and there are good indicators of a nice, gentle simmer.

4. Strain

Turn the heat off and let the broth cool for a few hours. In the middle of winter, I'll put my stockpot outside to cool it down more quickly. If there's snow on the ground, I'll put it right in the snow. Another option is to make an ice bath in your sink. Once cooled, remove the bones with a slotted spoon. Line a colander with cheesecloth or use a fine mesh strainer and strain the broth into another large bowl or another stockpot. Ladle the broth into your storage containers and let them cool in your kitchen a few more hours. If you're filling glass jars that will be stored in the freezer, always leave a few inches of headspace at the top of the jar. Broth will expand when frozen and can crack glass jars if they're overfilled.

5. Store

Store whatever you'll use for the week in your fridge. A layer of fat will form on top of the broths, which will act like a seal and preserve your broth for up to seven days in the fridge. Freeze the rest for long-term storage.

With that formula, let's apply it to the most basic types of broths.

Chapter 11

The Two Most Common Broths

Alright, here we go! Let's start with making the two most common broths: chicken and beef. I'd say 90 percent of recipes you'll find for soups will use one of these two broths. Now, if this is the first time you've made a homemade broth, I know it can be a little intimidating. As a reminder, my online course, How to Make Bone Broth 101, will give you some great visuals of the five-step formula as well as the different types of bones and animal parts to use for these broths. If at any point you feel you need a little more clarity, just head on over to www.HowToMakeBoneBroth101.com.

Chicken Broth

Ingredients

Yield – about 4 quarts

- 1 whole raw chicken (or raw whole chicken parts, cut up) or 1–2 chicken carcasses from a roasted chicken, meat removed
- Vegetables, coarsely chopped—2–3 carrots 2–3 stalks celery, 1 medium to large onion
- 2–4 Tbsp apple cider vinegar
- Filtered water to cover chicken

Optional chicken parts for more gelatin and nutrition

- 1–2 chicken backs
- 1–2 chicken feet
- Giblets (but not the liver)—these include the neck, heart, and gizzards
- Chicken head (often included on whole birds from ethnic markets)

Directions

- Step 1. Soak. Place chicken and/or chicken carcasses and parts in bottom of stockpot, cover with water, and add vinegar. Let sit for 30–60 minutes.
- Step 2. Skim. Bring to a gentle rolling boil and skim any scum that forms on the surface. Add veggies after skimming.
- Step 3. Simmer. Turn temperature to low and simmer very gently, covered, for 4–24 hours.
- Step 4. Strain. Let broth cool to about room temperature. Strain broth from bones, parts, and veggies and transfer to storage containers.
- Step 5. Store. Store in fridge for up to 7 days. Freeze whatever you won't use within a week.

Tips and Variations

1. For a larger batch of broth, use a larger stockpot and to the above ingredients add an extra whole chicken or an extra carcass or two and/or more chicken parts. Add additional veggies. Adjust the amount of water as needed.

2. Raw bones or previously cooked bones are equally good to use. Those with meat on them will add a nice depth of flavor. But if all you have are chicken bones that you've saved in your freezer, that's perfectly fine to use too! Add in some additional chicken parts (necks, backs, etc.) if you have them.

3. If using a whole, raw chicken or raw chicken parts with lots of meat on them, you can remove the chicken after about 3–5 hours and remove the meat from the bones. It should be well cooked and very tender. Reserve the meat for chicken salad or for a wonderful chicken soup. Return bones to the water and continue simmering.

4. If you're short on time, you can certainly make a lighter broth and simmer everything for just an hour or two. It won't have the depth of nutrition a longer-cooked broth contains, but it still beats the boxed stuff any day of the week!

5. Adding fresh herbs in the last 15–20 minutes of the simmering imparts additional minerals and flavors. Parsley and thyme are two common additions.

6. When the stock cools, a layer of fat will form on the surface. Despite what every fat-phobic recipe on the Internet says, don't skim it off! It will act as a seal and keep your stock fresher in the fridge for a longer period. When you do break the seal, you can either save the fat for use in other recipes (gravies, sautéing, etc.) or dissolve it back into the broth. Dissolving it back is a matter of personal preference. It will make your broth a little heavier. Perhaps wonderful for a cold winter night but not so much for other uses. You can also feed it to your dog, who will love you for it! The same applies for beef broth.

7. Sub turkey or duck carcasses in place of chicken. Or use a combination of different types of poultry bones.
8. For a pork broth, simply use pork bones instead of chicken. Pork broth is common in Asian cuisine and has a fairly neutral flavor. Use any pork bones you want in any combination—neck bones, leg bones, hocks, spareribs, etc. A mix of meaty bones and gelatinous bones is ideal. A gelatinous pig's foot is a great addition if you can find one. How to Make Bone Broth 101 includes a video for making pork broth with pigs' feet (which is always optional)!

Beef Broth

Ingredients

Yield – about 4 quarts

- 2–3 marrow bones
- 1–2 meaty bones like rib bones, shanks, and/or neck bones
- 1–2 large knuckle bones (These can be quite large and contain lots of gelatin. Usually one is all that will fit in an eight-quart stockpot.)

Vegetables, coarsely chopped –

- 2–3 carrots
- 2–3 stalks celery
- 1 medium to large onion

Herbs, optional –

- 3–4 sprigs thyme
- 1–2 bay leaves
- 1–2 tsp peppercorns
- ¼–½ cup apple cider vinegar
- Filtered water to cover

Optional beef parts for more gelatin and nutrition -

- 1 oxtail (an oxtail is the tail of the cow)
- 1 calf's foot

Directions

- Step 1. Soak. Place bones in stockpot, cover with water, and add vinegar. Let sit 30–60 minutes.
- Though not necessary, to develop more flavor, you can roast the meaty bones first. Brush with olive oil, set in a roasting pan, and roast at 350°F–400°F for about 40–60 minutes, until bones are browned but not charred. Then add to stockpot with other bones. You can also roast the veggies with the meaty bones too.
- Step 2. Skim. Bring to a boil and skim scum that rises to the surface. Add veggies after skimming.
- Step 3. Simmer. Reduce heat to a very gentle simmer. Add herbs and peppercorns. Simmer, covered, 12–72 hours.
- Step 4. Strain. Let broth cool to about room temperature. Remove larger bones with a slotted spoon. Strain broth and transfer to storage containers.
- Step 5. Store. Store in fridge for up to 7 days. Freeze whatever you won't use within a week.

Tips and Variations

1. Use whatever combination of bones you can get. The bones listed in the ingredients are recommended but not absolute. If all you have are a shank bone and a few marrow bones, good enough! Always save bones from other cuts like rib eyes and T-bones and add them to your beef broths. All of them will impart valuable minerals and nutrients.

2. If you're uncomfortable leaving your stove or Crock-Pot on overnight, simply turn it off before bed. It will still be warm in the morning. Bring the broth back to a boil and return to a gentle simmer.

3. For some great flavor variations, try adding a handful or two of dried mushrooms with the veggies. Another common addition is a cup of a dry, full-bodied red wine like Cabernet or Zinfandel.

4. I usually simmer beef broth in the 24–48 hour range. The only time I do 72 hours is when I come to the end of day two and I'm too tired to strain it out. So I let it go another day. Seventy-two hours is certainly a long time, so don't feel like you have to go that long. But you can!

5. Because beef bones are so thick, I always reuse the bones for a second batch of broth. I won't always do this immediately. I'll often keep the bones in the fridge for a day or two until I'm ready. The second batch won't be as gelatinous, but it will still be great. I've noticed recently that prices for bones are rising as they come more into demand for making broths. So a second batch is a great way to get more value! You can do this with chicken too if you've only simmered the chicken for a brief time.

6. Here's a great tip if you have a dog. For a simple and healthy (and free!) dog snack, when you strain the broth, save all the meat scraps, bone marrow, and fat and put it in a glass container in the fridge. (Be careful as you're doing this to not include any little pieces of bones as cooked bones can be dangerous for dogs.) This will form

a rather grotesque looking gelatinous mass. But your dog will LOVE it. It's like meat candy for dogs. Cut off pieces throughout the week and stuff them in a Kong toy (a rubber toy for dogs that is hollow in the middle). Your dog will be in heaven for the next half hour trying to lick, chew, and scrape every last bit out of the toy. My golden retriever, Lipton, and I will actually show you how to do this in How to Make Bone Broth 101.

7. As with the chicken broth, save the fat that congeals at the surface with cooling.

8. Sub lamb, goat, bison, and/or other wild game like venison for beef bones.

9. Double or even triple the ingredient amounts in a large stockpot for larger batches of broth. I mostly use a twenty-quart stockpot for beef broth these days.

Leftover Bones Broth

About once every two to three months, I'll make a bone broth from leftover bones that I've saved from different cuts of meat. These are often a combination of raw and cooked bones, but mostly cooked. I keep them in my freezer until I have enough to fill up a standard-sized stockpot that will get me about four quarts of broth.

The bones I save have little meat on them, they're not very gelatinous, and they're always a mix of different animal bones— chicken, turkey, beef, pork, and lamb.

I'll also throw in veggie scraps that I've saved as well—ends of carrots and onions, herb stems, kale stalks, beet greens, etc. And I'll usually chop up a few fresh ones as well. I'll also save some eggshells and add them for a little mineral boost.

I'll usually only simmer it for an hour or two and then use it for a soup I'm making that day. This broth doesn't gel, it's not too nutrient-rich, and it's rather flat tasting. Doesn't matter. Add a little salt and pepper, and it tastes delicious.

Ingredients

Yield – about 4 quarts

- 3–4 pounds leftover bones from beef, chicken, turkey, pork, lamb, etc.
- A few pounds vegetable scraps or fresh chopped vegetables—onions, carrots, celery, leeks, etc.
- 2–4 Tbsp apple cider vinegar
- Eggshells, optional
- Filtered water to cover

Directions

- Step 1. Soak. Put all ingredients in a stockpot and cover with water, and add vinegar. Let sit for 30–60 minutes.
- Step 2. Skim. Bring to a boil and skim scum that rises to the surface. Add veggies after skimming.
- Step 3. Simmer. Simmer gently for as long as you can.
- Step 4. Strain. Strain broth and transfer to storage containers.
- Step 5. Store. Store in fridge for up to 7 days. Freeze whatever you won't use within a week.

Chapter 12

The Cheapest and Quickest Broth

I'm talking about fish broth! Fish broth is my absolute favorite broth, and I consider it a great tragedy that so few people make homemade fish broth anymore. Without question, it is the *cheapest and quickest* broth to make.

All you need for fish broth is a good source of fish carcasses. Your local fishmonger, commercial fisherman, or even the seafood department at your local supermarket will give them to you for practically nothing because so few people value them anymore. Once the fish are fileted, they just throw out the carcasses. What a waste!

You'll want the carcasses from non-oily whitefish like cod, sole, snapper, haddock, and hake. Any non-oily fish works fine. The delicate fats in oily fish like salmon, tuna, herring, and swordfish don't stand up well to heat and thus don't work well for fish broth (though their flesh works great in chowders and other fish-based soups).

Generally speaking, you probably won't get much gelatin from fish carcasses. Gelatin-rich fish heads, though, prized throughout Asia, are another story. They're also a good source of iodine, a trace mineral that plays vital roles in endocrine health (especially thyroid health), which many Americans are deficient in. Ask your local sources to throw in some extra fish heads with the carcasses.

The great thing about fish broth, besides the flavor, is that the delicate oils only need a short simmer time to infuse the broth with a wonderful fish essence. All you need is an hour! For that reason, the first step in the five-step formula is a little different with fish broth. Instead of soaking the fish carcasses, which is not really necessary, the first step is to dice the veggies fine and sauté them in some butter for about five to ten minutes. This will help them better release their flavors with the shorter simmer time. After five to ten minutes, the fish carcasses are then added and simmered another five to ten minutes over the veggies. This also helps to stimulate the fish carcasses to release their flavors before adding the water. The next four steps in the five-step formula are the same.

White wine and herbs are other common additions. Though optional, they can make a big difference with the shorter simmer time, so I do recommend them. How to Make Bone Broth 101 definitely includes a video for fish broth!

Fish Broth

Ingredients

Yield – about 4 quarts

- 1–2 non-oily fish carcasses from cod, sole, haddock, hake, etc.
- 1 Tbsp butter
- Vegetables, diced fine – 1 onion, 1–2 carrots, 1–2 stalks celery
- 1 cup dry white wine, optional
- Herbs, optional – 3–4 sprigs thyme, 2 bay leaves, ½–1 tsp peppercorns
- Filtered water to cover

For extra gelatin

- 1–2 fish heads, gills removed

Directions

- Step 1. Simmer veggies in butter and white wine over medium heat for about 5–10 minutes. Place fish carcasses, fish heads (if using), herbs, and peppercorns over veggies, cover and simmer 5–10 more minutes.
- Step 2. Skim. Add water to cover bones, bring to a simmer, and skim scum.
- Step 3. Simmer. Simmer for about 1 hour.
- Step 4. Strain. Strain broth from carcasses and veggies.
- Step 5. Store. Store in fridge for up to 5 days. Freeze whatever you won't use within that time.

Tips and Variations

10. For a more gelatinous fish broth, use a few pounds of fish heads in place of the fish carcasses.
11. Double up the amounts in a larger stockpot.
12. Try other herbs—parsley, fennel, cloves, etc. all work well.

Chapter 13

Big Idea #3 for Making Broths

This is one final big idea to keep in mind when making bone broths. And it should be noted that this big idea applies mostly to chicken and beef broths. As previously discussed, a sign of a good bone broth is how well it gels due to the presence of gelatin. Upon cooling, the broth should giggle like Jell-O. But don't worry if that doesn't happen. The best piece of advice I ever heard was from Shannon Hayes, farmer and cookbook author, who said, "Don't you dare throw out that broth if it doesn't gel!" And that is big idea #3 for making broths.

There are a few reasons your broth may not gel. First, as mentioned above, quality and variety matter. People have reported that conventional bones and animal parts don't gel well. And of course, the more gelatinous bones and parts you use, the more likely you'll get a rich, gelatinous broth. But again, it can be hard to find things like chicken feet and oxtails, so don't stress if all you have is a chicken carcass. Good enough!

The second reason is time. You won't get much gelatin if you only simmer things for an hour. But if that's all the time you have, well, again, that's OK!

Third, adding too much water can dilute the gelatin. A good rule of thumb is about one to two pounds of bones per quart of water. Another way to gauge this is to fill your pot about half full with bones and animal parts and then cover everything with water.

And fourth, boiling broths for too long can also prevent gelatin from forming. As previously discussed, broths should be very gently simmered. A good gauge of a gentle simmer is a few bubbles rising to the surface here and there. Even a rolling boil is too high of a temperature. If you're cooking on a stove top, that would mean a fairly low temperature setting. This is why I don't recommend Crock-Pots. Most Crock-Pots' lowest temperature setting is too high and will boil the broth.

Taking all this into account, creating gelatin in broths can still be a little hit or miss. Sometimes I get a lot of gelatin and sometimes I get hardly any. Most people I know who make broths regularly say the same thing.

Finally, gelatin is great for many health issues, but not everyone wants tons of gelatin in their broths. Some people with underlying digestive problems, such as gallbladder issues, have a hard time digesting gelatinous broths. If that describes you, it's OK to simmer your broths for a shorter time period.

You can also add water to gelatinous broths upon reheating to thin them out.

PART III

FEARLESS BROTH FOR BREAKFAST

Chapter 14

8 Reasons You Should Have Broth for Breakfast

When I tell people I have bone broth for breakfast, I could just as well tell them I have monkey brains for breakfast. The reaction is pretty much the same—part shock and part confusion. I know broth is not exactly a staple breakfast food in America, but let me give you eight reasons you should have broths for breakfast:

Reason #1: They're great when you're in a rush.

Warm up some broth. Add in whatever you want—some greens, some chopped garlic, poach some eggs in there, maybe throw in some leftover chicken or sausage, spice it up with salt and pepper or soy sauce. Boom. Breakfast is ready in five minutes.

Reason #2: They're light yet nourishing.

I hear this all the time: "But I'm not hungry in the morning." Many people don't do well with heavier protein-based breakfasts for many reasons. They often skip breakfast as a result but regret it a few hours later when they're starving at work and have nothing prepared.

If you're one of those people who get nauseous at the thought of eggs and bacon in the morning, consider having broths for breakfast instead. They're easily digestible and won't make you feel bloated. But if you're like me and need a bit more protein…

Reason #3: You can still have eggs!

Broths don't have to be light. If you're one of those who thrive on heartier breakfasts, broths can still do the trick. Adding a good protein and some starch like rice or potatoes can make for a very filling meal. And the easiest way to add some quick protein is to add some eggs. They work well in almost any broth. You can poach 'em right in the broth, and they'll cook in just a few minutes. Add 'em whole or just add the yolks.

Reason #4: You can still have oatmeal!

Millions start their day with sweetened oatmeal topped with overly sweetened yogurt, but you can actually have a savory oatmeal with bone broth instead. That may, once again, sound as enticing as eating monkey brains, but I challenge you to try one of the savory oatmeal recipes that follow. I can almost guarantee you'll love it. Sure, it's a little outside the box of a typical American breakfast, but this book is not about being inside the box. I hope that's obvious by now. Speaking of boxes…

Reason #5: They're healthier than boxed breakfast cereal.

Standard of all standard American breakfasts, nothing beats convenience more than boxed breakfast cereal. But few people realize that boxed breakfast cereals, including whole grain organic ones, go through a high-tech process known as "extrusion." It's a high heat, high pressure process that creates all those flakes and shapes and it's been shown to damage the nutrient content.[4]

Furthermore, despite the popular mantra to "eat more whole grains," grains can be hard to digest. Whole grains have a protective outer shell called the bran that keeps the nutrients tightly locked inside. Traditionally, cultures would soak, sprout,

---

[4] Sally Fallon Morell, "Dirty Secrets of the Food Processing Industry," *Weston A. Price Foundation*, December 26, 2005, http://www.westonaprice.org/health-topics/dirty-secrets-of-the-food-processing-industry/.

and ferment grains, which helps to release the bran and make them more digestible. Even Quaker Oats used to include instructions on their label for soaking oats overnight. These traditional practices slowly faded in favor of quick, highly processed grain-based cereals. As a result, many people are unknowingly eating tons of improperly prepared grains with tons of sugar. Nothing more exemplifies this than boxed breakfast cereals.

Reason #6: It's cold outside.

What sounds like a better way to start out your day on a *bone-chillingly* cold winter morning? Cold breakfast cereal or a steaming bowl of nourishing broth? I rest my case.

Reason #7: They're just as good for lunch or dinner.

There are eighteen simple breakfast recipes in the next three chapters—five with broth and eggs, seven with oatmeal, and six with rice (congee). It doesn't get any easier than these. But you don't have to make them just for breakfast! They're all perfectly suited to other meals of the day as well. When I come home after a long day and the thought of cooking makes me more exhausted than I already am, it's nice to know I can whip up any of these recipes for a quick and simple dinner.

Reason #8: You'll get bonus recipes!

I had so much fun experimenting with these breakfast recipes that I wound up with *a lot* more than I could include here. I've made some of the extras available as free bonus downloads on my website. There are a few bonus recipes for each chapter below (including the soup chapters in Part IV), and you can download them all on one PDF here:
http://www.fearlesseating.net/fearless-broths-and-soups-bonus-recipes.

Chapter 15

Broth for Breakfast: Broth and Eggs

The recipes below follow three very simple steps. First, bring your broth to a simmer. Second, add veggies and eggs and simmer a few minutes. Third, add seasonings to taste. That's it! To make things more ample, serve with a side of sourdough toast and butter and/or include some precooked rice or potatoes in the second step. Finally, all of these recipes are for one bowl of broth at 1–2 cups with 1–2 eggs. Adjust amounts and ingredients as needed.

Basic Eggs in Broth

Ingredients

- 1–2 cups broth of choice
- 1–2 eggs
- Grated Parmesan cheese
- Several sprigs parsley, chopped
- Salt and pepper, to taste

Directions

1. Bring broth to a simmer.
2. Add in eggs and simmer a few minutes, until whites are cooked but yolks are still soft and runny.
3. Top with Parmesan cheese, parsley, and salt and pepper, to taste.

Tips and Variations

1. Poached eggs will look a bit messy in the broth. The ends of the whites will fray and loosely float around. If you like your food to look pretty, here's a little trick: before you add in the eggs, swirl the simmering broth with a kitchen utensil in a clockwise direction. Then drop in the eggs and continue swirling for about a minute. The egg whites will fold around the yolk and form a more rounded shape. I will often do this for my own entertainment. Nice looking or not, it will all taste the same, which is delicious, of course!

Basic Eggs in Broth, Asian-Style

Ingredients

- 1–2 cups broth of choice
- 1–2 eggs
- 1–2 cloves garlic, chopped
- 1-inch piece of ginger, chopped
- Kale, chopped
- Soy sauce or fish sauce, to taste

Directions

1. Bring broth to a simmer, add in ginger and garlic, and simmer a few more minutes, longer if you have time, to further infuse garlic and ginger flavor.
2. Add in eggs and kale and simmer a few minutes, until eggs are cooked and kale is thoroughly wilted.
3. Season to taste with soy sauce or fish sauce.

Tips and Variations

1. If time allows, sauté the ginger and garlic in some olive, sesame, or coconut oil for a few minutes and then add them into the broth. This will release the flavors a little better than just plopping them in after the broth is simmering.
2. Add in some chili peppers or hot sauce for an extra kick.
3. Add in a drizzle or two of sesame oil at the end.

Eggs in a Tomato-Basil Broth with Sausage

Ingredients

- 1–2 cups chicken or beef broth
- 1–2 eggs
- 1 tsp tomato paste
- ¼–½ link sausage, crumbled or chopped into circles
- 3–4 basil leaves, chopped
- Salt and pepper, to taste

Directions

1. Bring broth to a simmer. Remove about ½ cup to a bowl, mix in tomato paste, and return to the broth, mixing thoroughly.
2. Add sausage and cook about 1 minute. Add in eggs and poach a few minutes.
3. Top with basil and season to taste with salt and pepper.

Tips and Variations

1. Add a little more or less tomato paste, to your liking.
2. Sub diced tomatoes, canned or fresh, for the tomato paste
3. If you have time, sauté the sausage separately in oil for more flavor and then add it to the broth at the end. Or, leave out the sausage entirely.

Miso Soup

You're probably familiar with the miso soup that's often served as an appetizer in Japanese restaurants. There are two basic ingredients. The first is miso, which is just a fermented soybean paste that is readily available in most health food stores. There are usually several types of miso paste, the most common ones being red miso and white miso. Use whatever you like. Personally, I like the darker red miso pastes, which are fermented longer and are a bit saltier and more strongly flavored.

The second basic ingredient is the broth. Traditionally, miso soup uses a light broth known as "dashi," which is made from dried bonito flakes. But any broth can be used as a substitute. Fish broth in particular works really well.

The great thing about miso soup is that all you need to do is add miso paste to the broth and you have an instant soup. After that, you can add in almost anything you want. It's just a matter of personal preference, and it all comes together in just a matter of minutes. This is also why it makes such a great breakfast!

Ingredients

- 1–2 cups broth of choice
- 1–2 tsp miso paste
- 1–2 eggs
- Tofu, cut into cubes, optional
- 1 scallion, chopped
- Soy sauce, optional

Directions

1. Bring broth to a simmer. Remove ¼ cup to a bowl, mix in miso paste, and return to the broth, mixing thoroughly.
2. Add eggs and tofu and simmer until eggs are poached.
3. Top with scallions. Season to taste with soy sauce, if needed.

Tips and Variations

The above recipe is about as basic as it gets. There are a million ways to vary things up. Below are five super simple, three-ingredient recipes that you can add to the base of miso and broth. Eggs can be substituted for any of the proteins. Or added with them. Or excluded. Totally up to you.

1. Shrimp, bok choy, and Sriracha
2. Fish, mushrooms, and napa cabbage
3. Chicken, rice, leftover carrots, and/or broccoli
4. Pork, scallions, spinach
5. Beef, string beans, parsley

Egg Drop Soup

Ingredients

- 1–2 cups chicken broth
- 1–2 eggs, beaten in separate bowl or cup
- Chives or scallions
- Salt and pepper, to taste
- Hot sauce, to taste, optional

Directions

1. Bring broth to a simmer.
2. In a slow and steady stream, pour in the egg mixture. Continue to stir the egg mixture around in the broth for a minute or two, until the eggs form thin strands.
3. Top with chives or scallions and season to taste with salt and pepper and optional hot sauce.

Want more broth-for-breakfast recipes?

Download them for free here:

http://www.fearlesseating.net/fearless-broths-and-soups-bonus-recipes

Chapter 16

Broth for Breakfast: Savory Oatmeal

The first time I heard about savory oatmeal, I was suspicious. A friend of mine e-mailed me her savory oatmeal recipe and at first glance, I thought, "Bone broth? In oatmeal? Dear God... NO!"

After all, oatmeal is *supposed to be sweet*. Everyone knows that. Like the sky is up. Like dogs are better than cats (sorry, cat lovers). And like bacon is the greatest food ever. It's just a law of nature.

Then again, who would've thought butter and coconut oil go so well in coffee? If you have not yet heard about this phenomenon, just Google "bulletproof coffee." And then try it. The first time I did I was hooked, and that's the exact same experience I had with savory oatmeal.

Savory oatmeal has now become a regular in my breakfast repertoire, especially in the winter. I'll even have it on occasion for lunch or dinner. It's a quick and nourishing meal that can be had at any time of the day.

How to Make Savory Oatmeal in Three Simple Steps:

1. 1. Soak one part oatmeal to two parts warm water, along with a tablespoon of whey, yogurt, or lemon juice, overnight in your kitchen. This will make the oatmeal more digestible and able to be cooked up very quickly.
2. 2. In the morning, strain soaking water and add 1–2 cups chicken or beef broth and a chopped clove of garlic and simmer for about 5 minutes.
3. 3. Season to taste with salt or soy sauce and any type of hot sauce you like. Other possibilities include Worcestershire sauce, coconut aminos, or fish sauce.
4. That's it!

Of course, that's a little plain (though still delicious). You can liven things up by adding all sorts of veggies, herbs, spices, and even nuts and different meats. And eggs ALWAYS work well in savory oatmeal. Add a hard-boiled egg, a fried egg, or poach an egg in the broth while simmering.

Seven Super Simple Savory Oatmeal Recipes

Here are seven ridiculously easy recipes to take savory oatmeal to the next level . . . so easy that ingredient lists aren't even necessary!

Savory Oatmeal with a Fried Egg and Sriracha

This is the first recipe I learned from my friend. Eggs in oatmeal may sound a little strange, but just give it a chance. I'm certain you'll be pleasantly surprised. And if Sriracha doesn't float your boat, just leave it out.

Directions

Simmer oatmeal with a clove or two of chopped garlic. Add a drizzle of Worcestershire sauce and top with a fried egg (or two). Add salt and pepper and Sriracha, to taste.

Tips and Variations

1. Add some chopped chilies for some extra spiciness.
2. Add some kimchi.
3. Top with some cilantro or parsley.

Savory Oatmeal with Peas and Peanuts

When I was in Burma, another common breakfast besides mohinga was a simple plate of boiled rice with peas and peanuts. Sounds a bit dull, I know, but for whatever reason, peas and peanuts complement each other beautifully. A drizzle of sesame oil and salt rounds this out into pea-nutty perfection.

Directions

Add frozen or fresh peas in the last 2 minutes to the simmering oatmeal. Top with peanuts and a drizzle of sesame oil (optional). Season to taste with salt.

Tips and Variations

1. Add soy sauce or fish sauce.
2. Add Sriracha or any other hot sauce.
3. Top with some lightly sautéed mushrooms, onions, and/or garlic.

Extra Savory Oatmeal with Mushrooms, Parmesan, and Chives

This is *hands down* my favorite savory oatmeal recipe. The mushrooms and Parmesan make this recipe extra savory and give it a slight resemblance to a creamy mushroom risotto.

Directions

To simmering oatmeal, add mushrooms. When ready, mix in grated Parmesan, season with salt, and top with fresh chives.

Tips and Variations

1. Sauté the mushrooms separately in some oil for a richer flavor.
2. If sautéing mushrooms, throw in some diced red onion.
3. Sub scallions in place of chives. Or add both!
4. Sub soy sauce for salt.
5. Top with a fried egg.

Bacon-Avocado-Egg Savory Oatmeal

This one is so good that you may want to send me thank-you gifts as a token of your appreciation. I won't object.

Directions

Sauté the bacon and egg separately. Add with the avocado when oatmeal is done. Season to taste with salt.

Tips and Variations

1. Add in some chopped tomato.
2. Throw in some chopped scallions with the bacon.
3. Leave out the bacon entirely (though you won't be as inclined to send me gifts).

Savory Oatmeal with Cashews and Nori Strips

Very Japanese and very delicious.

Directions

When oatmeal is done simmering, top with cashews and strips of nori, and season to taste with soy sauce.

Tips and Variations

1. Top with a drizzle of sesame oil (highly recommended).
2. Top with some cilantro or scallions. Or both!
3. Sub peanuts for cashews.

Savory Oatmeal with Kale and Soy Sauce

Not sure what the big hysteria is these days over kale? Me either. But kale in bone broth is another story. Let's face it, kale and other leafy greens are inherently bitter. They need to be combined with other foods and softened with some heat to make them more palatable and digestible. A perfect vehicle for that is broth!

Directions

Add kale while oatmeal is simmering. Season to taste with soy sauce.

Tips and Variations

1. Drizzle with sesame oil.
2. Add Sriracha or hot sauce of choice.
3. Add a hard-boiled egg or two for some additional protein.

Savory Oatmeal with Sausage, Onions, and Peppers

Here's a simple way to come up with additional savory oatmeal recipes: if it works in an omelet, it will probably work in savory oatmeal. This is a good example of that.

Directions

Chop the sausage, onions, and peppers and add at the beginning of simmering until cooked. This will only take a few minutes. Alternatively, sauté them separately and mix in when oatmeal is done. Season to taste with salt and pepper.

Tips and Variations

1. Top with a sunny-side up egg.
2. Season with hot sauce.
3. Add rosemary, sage, and/or thyme.

Want more savory oatmeal recipes?

Download them for free here:

http://www.fearlesseating.net/fearless-broths-and-soups-bonus-recipes

Chapter 17

Broth for Breakfast: Congee

Congee is basically the oatmeal of Asia. But instead of oats, it's made with rice. The rice is cooked in broth for an extended time, which breaks it down and turns it into a porridge-like consistency. From that simple foundation almost anything can be added, and the bewildering variety of congee dishes across Asia is a testament to its versatility.

Prepared at home from fresh ingredients and your own homemade bone broth, congee is a perfect example of a meal that is not only healthy, but cheap too. In fact, it's commonly considered food for the poor in Asia. But keep in mind that at one time, lobster was considered food for the poor too. Considering the recent craze over bone broth, congee may very well become the next pricey food trend here in the United States. Even more reason to learn to make it at home before you have to shell out top dollar for it!

But the best thing about congee is that it's easy to cook it in bulk, so you can easily prepare a week's worth of congee at once.

How to Make Congee in Three Simple Steps:

Step 1: Cook the rice in the broth.

First, rinse the rice in water a few times to wash away extra starch, which could make the congee too thick and starchy.

Next, decide on the amount of broth and rice you're going to use. The ratio of the broth to the rice and the length of time you cook it will determine its consistency and texture. There's no absolute rule for this. It just depends how you like it. It may also take some experimentation to find what you like.

For a cup of white rice, add anywhere from 2–4 quarts of broth. Generally speaking, you want to cook the rice for about 1–1 ½ hours. At that time, 2 quarts of broth will give a fairly thick consistency similar to oatmeal and 4 quarts will be more like the consistency of soup. Personally, I prefer the latter.

Now remember, we're not cooking a side of fluffy, tender rice here, so don't be afraid to cook this until the rice starts to break apart and lose its shape. You may even go as long as 2–2 ½ hours. Just keep an eye on it until you get the desired texture and consistency.

And don't worry if it turns out too thick or thin. You can always readjust the consistency by adding more broth to thin it out or cooking it down to thicken it further.

To cook the rice, bring the broth to a boil and then reduce the heat and cook at a rolling boil, stirring on occasion to prevent sticking. Keep the lid on the pot but leave it slightly ajar to let steam escape.

An Important Tip

Just a heads-up. The ratios above will make A LOT of congee. You may want to start out with less. Totally fine. But eventually, I would recommend making a larger amount at once. Obviously, you're not going to simmer a bowl of congee for an hour every morning. Do it once on the weekend and you'll have an instant breakfast (or lunch or dinner!) all week long. How's that for convenience?

Also, because this larger batch is essentially just rice cooked in broth, you can then transfer single servings to a separate pot and then use steps 2–4 below to create a wide variety of different recipes.

Once you have the rice ready, everything else comes together *very quickly*.

Step 2: Add protein and vegetables.

Almost any type of vegetable will work in a congee. Some vegetables you may want to sauté separately in some oil to bring out more depth of flavor. It's totally up to you. Usually, time is what dictates what I'll add. If I'm in a rush, I plop everything in the broth and simmer for a few minutes. If I have a little more time, I might cook up some veggies separately.

The same could be said for different proteins. Congees work well with all types of meats as well as eggs.

Step 3: Add herbs, seasonings, and spices.

This is where the congee magic really happens. Salt, soy sauce, fish sauce, and Sriracha are common additions that instantly transform a rather plain-tasting congee into something bursting with flavor.

As for herbs, it's hard to go wrong with things like cilantro, chives, parsley, thyme, and oregano.

The choices are almost infinite.

Experiment!

Optional Step 4: Top with fried garlic, scallions, and/or shallots and onions.

This is optional, but I HIGHLY recommend it as it works in almost any congee recipe. Fry until browned and crispy but not blackened. These will add not only a nice crunch to complement the congee but also some wonderful smoky flavors too.

Six Simple Three-Step Congee Recipes

For all of these recipes, the serving size is for one bowl. For one serving, transfer already prepared congee from step 1 above to a separate pot for heating and/or adding ingredients. Adjust serving size as needed.

After that, you're just three short steps away from a beautiful bowl of congee heaven.

Also, it's implied that every recipe will be greatly enhanced by adding some fried garlic and scallions or shallots/onions!

Asian Chicken Congee

Ingredients

- 1 bowl congee cooked in chicken broth
- 1-inch piece of ginger, peeled and chopped
- 1–2 cloves garlic, chopped
- 1 Thai red chili, de-seeded and chopped, optional
- Handful cooked, shredded chicken
- 1 scallion, chopped
- Soy sauce, to taste

Optional Accompaniments

- Fresh cilantro, chopped
- Sesame oil, to taste
- Sriracha, to taste
- Lemon wedge

Directions

- Step 1. Add ginger, garlic, and optional chili to congee and simmer for 5–10 minutes.
- Step 2. Add chicken and scallions and simmer a minute or two.
- Step 3. Season to taste with soy sauce. Add optional accompaniments.

Sweet Potato Coconut Curry Congee

Ingredients

- 1 bowl congee cooked in chicken (preferred) or beef broth
- Coconut milk, a dollop to a ¼ cup
- ½ tsp–1 tsp curry powder
- Sweet potatoes, cooked and chopped into bite-sized pieces
- Fresh, chopped tomatoes, optional
- Salt, to taste

Directions

- Step 1. Add coconut milk and curry powder to congee and simmer a few minutes. Add more coconut milk and curry powder to taste.
- Step 2. Add sweet potatoes and optional tomatoes and cook a few minutes. If using uncooked sweet potatoes, simmer about 10–15 minutes, until cooked through. Add more broth, if needed.
- Step 3. Salt to taste.

Ginger-Scallion Pork Congee

Ingredients

- 1 bowl congee cooked in chicken or pork broth
- 1-inch piece of ginger, peeled and diced
- Handful cooked pork, shredded or chopped
- 1–2 scallions, chopped
- Soy sauce, to taste

Directions

- Step 1. Bring congee to a simmer, add ginger, and simmer 5–10 minutes.
- Step 2. Add pork and scallions and simmer a few minutes more.
- Step 3. Add soy sauce to taste.

Crumbled Sausage with Thyme Congee

Ingredients

- 1 bowl congee cooked in chicken or beef broth
- ½–1 sausage, removed from casing and crumbled
- A few sprigs fresh thyme or 1 tsp dried thyme
- 1 egg, optional
- Sriracha or other hot sauce, to taste, optional
- Salt, to taste

Directions

1. Bring congee to a simmer, add crumbled sausage and thyme, and cook a few minutes, until sausage is cooked through.
2. Add in egg and poach in liquid a few minutes (optional).
3. Add salt and optional hot sauce to taste.

Rosemary Turkey Congee

Ingredients

- 1 bowl congee cooked in chicken or turkey broth
- Handful cooked turkey meat or 1 whole leftover turkey wing
- Sweet potatoes, previously cooked and chopped
- Handful spinach, optional
- 1 tsp fresh or dried rosemary
- Salt, to taste

Directions

1. Bring congee to a simmer, add turkey meat or whole wing, and simmer a few minutes.
2. Add optional spinach and rosemary and simmer a few more minutes.
3. Season to taste with salt.

Shrimp and Scallion Congee

Ingredients

- 1 bowl congee cooked in chicken broth
- 1–2 pieces scallions, chopped
- 1–2 cloves garlic, chopped
- 1-inch piece ginger, peeled and chopped
- Handful cooked or raw shrimp
- Fish sauce, to taste
- 1 lemon or lime wedge, optional

Directions

1. Bring congee to a simmer, add garlic, ginger, and scallions, and simmer 5–10 minutes.
2. Add shrimp and cook a few minutes (if raw).
3. Season to taste with fish sauce and lemon or lime.

Want more congee recipes?

Download them for free here:

http://www.fearlesseating.net/fearless-broths-and-soups-bonus-recipes

PART IV
FEARLESS SOUPS

Chapter 18

3 Simple Steps to Set You Free

In my opinion, the purpose of a good recipe book is to give you the skills to take those recipes and make them your own. It should leave room for experimentation so that you can adapt, tweak, and improvise different ingredients for different variations. Cooking is ultimately a creative endeavor!

Jessica Prentice, in *Full Moon Feast*, says:

> *"We are used to written recipes that are extremely precise, and we are used to following them exactly. But until a little over a century ago there were no such things as measuring cups or spoons. Recipes often gave some ideas as to measurement, but it was vague at best. The cook had to rely on her own judgment, skill, and, even more important, on her senses. She had to really look at the food, to watch it, to touch it, to smell it, to taste it, even to listen to it."[5]*

She goes on to say that *"I certainly read lots of recipes, but I very rarely (if ever) follow one exactly. It takes the creativity away."[6]*

Ultimately, that's what I hope this book will do for you. And this is why I'm a fan of coming up with simple step-by-step formulas and why I use them so often in this book. They serve

---

[5] Prentice, Full Moon Feast, 245.
[6] Ibid. 247.

as a springboard for creating your own recipes. This is especially true when it comes to making broth-based soups, because once you have homemade bone broths ready to go in your fridge and freezer, you are just three simple steps away from an infinite amount of simple soup creations. In the chapters that follow, you will see how this simple three-step formula is repeated over and over with all the different recipes. In time, you can use these three steps to come up with your own. And who knows, maybe someday you won't even need recipes anymore!

Here's the simple three-step formula:

Step 1. Sauté hard vegetables in butter or oil for 5–10 minutes.

"Hard" vegetables means any vegetables that need a little heat to soften. Those are usually vegetables like onions, garlic, carrots (and other root vegetables), celery, and leeks. This initial heating will also release their flavors and aromas and add more depth and complexity to your soup.

Step 2. Add broth, bring to a boil, and simmer another 5–10 minutes.

This step is pretty straightforward. You can often bring out more flavor in the vegetables by simmering them longer than 5–10 minutes. But I rarely do. If you're really in a rush, you can even combine steps 1 and 2. That is, heat the broth first and then throw in your harder vegetables. This is also the step where you would add starches like rice or potatoes and simmer them until softened.

Step 3. Add soft vegetables and soft meats, cook another 5–10 minutes, and season to taste.

"Soft" vegetables means any vegetables that only need a little heat to soften. That usually means greens like kale or spinach. And by "soft meats" I mean things like chicken, fish, and shellfish. They cook fairly quickly, usually anywhere from 2–5 minutes. Harder cuts of meat like tougher cuts of red meat are better for stews that need a longer cooking time to break down the strong fibers and connective tissue.

Additional Steps

For the most part, all of the recipes in Part IV will follow this three-step formula. Of course, it's not always that straightforward. Sometimes there are some additional steps. And sometimes there are less! But for the sake of simplicity, any additional steps will be grouped into the basic three steps. For example, in some of the recipes, additional ingredients are added after the hard vegetables and simmered a little longer. I'll include that all in step 1. Sometimes a few things happen after simmering the broth, like preparing noodles or adding potatoes or other vegetables. I'll group those together in step 2. Finally, adding garnishes and seasonings at the end is so minor that I include it in step 3. I hope that by keeping things grouped together in three steps, it will help you to keep things organized not only on paper but in your head too. There's nothing more intimidating than seeing a recipe that includes directions for twenty different steps!

Five Additional Recipe Tips:

1. Making soups in bulk means less time in the kitchen.

I shoot for using two quarts of broth for each recipe. Some recipes will only use a quart of broth because there's the addition of other things like coconut milk or cream. And some only use a quart because they're not easily adaptable to larger portion sizes. Regardless, those are good-sized portions and by making these soups in bulk, you'll save lots of time in the kitchen. If you're feeding a small family, you should get at least two leftover meals from the soups that are two quarts in size. If you're single, you'll have ready-made meals for just about every day of the week. And when you come home tired and don't feel like cooking, that's pretty awesome. By all means, use more or less broth and adjust the ingredients accordingly.

2. Soups are easy to adapt if you're on a special diet.

Some recipes use ingredients that are common food allergens or sensitivities like gluten, dairy, or corn. Many are easily adaptable by either deleting that ingredient or substituting another one. A few, however, such as the creamy vegetable soups that use dairy, are not. Where possible, I will recommend substitutions.

3. Use good-quality cooking fats.

I use only good-quality butter, olive oil, sesame oil, coconut oil, and lard. Yes, lard! Contrary to popular belief, animal fats are excellent for cooking because they're stable at high heat. At the risk of getting into a long discussion about good fats and bad fats, here's a good rule of thumb to follow: if it's been used in traditional cuisines for thousands of years, it's a good fat to use. Of course, modern processing can damage even good-quality fats, so be sure to seek out unrefined, good-quality products. Regardless, there are four you should avoid at all costs: canola, cottonseed, corn, and soybean. These are byproducts of industrial agriculture and have never been used for cooking purposes until the twentieth century. They are all highly refined and most are genetically modified.

4. Ingredient amounts are adjustable.

You'll see I often say "3–6 cloves garlic" or "1–2 Tbsp" of something. A little more or less of something is up to you and simply a matter of personal preference. Similarly, feel free to add ingredients or subtract some where you see fit. Don't be afraid to use your intuition and improvise! You'll be amazed at the things you come up with.

5. Two bonus recipes follow each chapter!

Similar to the broth for breakfast recipes, each chapter will include some free bonus recipes as well. You'll see the link after each chapter where you can download them for free on my website.

Chapter 19

Asian Noodle Soups

It was a trip to Thailand where I first fell in love with Asian noodle soups. Because they were made fresh every day, with local ingredients from Thai cooks (not chefs) who were *not* following written recipes, no two bowls of noodle soup ever tasted the same. Because of that, every meal for the entire four months of my trip had a little tinge of excitement. "What is THIS ONE going to taste like?" I would think to myself while waiting in eager anticipation for the meal to arrive.

I loved them all—the hot and sour soups, the mildly spicy red curries, the super spicy green curries, the sweet yellow (also called massaman) curries, all swimming in scents of fresh lemongrass, ginger, Thai basil, and fish sauce. And I loved that at every street stall and at every table in every café and restaurant there was a little caddy of sauces that you'd add to your personal taste. Fish sauce, soy sauce, chili garlic sauce, a sweet hoisin sauce, and a super spicy fermented chili pepper sauce (which once set my mouth on fire and left me sucking air for the next few hours) were the common denominators.

The beauty of Asian noodle soups is that the initial bowl of broth is usually just a starting point. So much of the final flavor depends on WHAT YOU LIKE. Most Asian noodle soups come with multiple accompaniments on the side—herbs like cilantro and basil, seasonings like soy sauce, lemon and lime wedges, fresh chilies, hot sauces, etc. You add as much or as little as you want. It makes creating these soups at home a lot of fun. And easy.

The recipes included here are just a small sampling but are a good starting point. I hope they inspire you to seek out additional recipes from different Asian countries! The possibilities are endless.

Types of Noodles

For the most part, you'll find a few different varieties sold in dried form in American supermarkets (especially health food stores), the most common ones being udon, soba, Chinese egg noodles, and rice noodles. Most noodles are either wheat-based or rice-based, and many now include blends of wheat and other grains. Asian supermarkets will have an often bewildering variety and sometimes will have freshly prepared noodles.

Here's what you need to know for this book:

1. Use whatever noodles you want in any of these recipes. They're all interchangeable.
2. Experiment with different types of noodles. They have a wide variety of textures, shapes, and subtle flavors.
3. Wheat-based noodles include udon and egg noodles. Udon is a thicker, chewier noodle and is especially tender if you can find it freshly made. Chinese egg noodles come in a wide variety of forms including lo mein, chow mein, and wonton.
4. Soba noodles are fairly thin noodles and are made from buckwheat, which gives them a pleasant nutty flavor. Buckwheat, despite its name, is not made from wheat. However, many soba noodles sold in stores are made from a blend of buckwheat and wheat. If you're on a gluten-free diet, be sure to check the label.
5. Rice noodles are very neutral tasting and will easily absorb the flavors of the soup. They're another good choice if you're gluten-free. They also come in a wide variety of shapes and sizes including an ultra-thin cut known as vermicelli.

6. If you're on a grain-free diet, you may be able to find some grain-free noodles made from mung beans. These are sometimes called "cellophane" or "glass" noodles. Similar versions are sometimes made from yams or other potato starches. Another grain-free noodle you might find is called "shirataki," which comes from an Asian root vegetable. Alternatively, you can just leave the noodles out entirely! All of these recipes will still work great without them.

7. Different noodles require different cooking times. Just follow the directions on the package.

8. Many noodles sold in both Asian supermarkets and conventional American supermarkets are highly processed. I've included a list of some good quality noodles on my broths and soups resources page:

http://fearlesseating.net/fearless-broths-and-soups-resources

Basic Asian Noodle Soup

I'm not sure there's ever been a more perfect match than ginger, garlic, broth, and fish sauce or soy sauce. This simple Asian noodle soup doesn't need much else. Add any meat your heart desires.

Ingredients

- 2 quarts bone broth—beef, chicken, fish, pork
- Any meat you like
- 1 Tbsp sesame, coconut, or olive oil
- 2–3-inch piece of ginger, diced
- 3–6 cloves garlic, diced
- Any greens you like
- Noodles of choice
- Soy sauce and/or fish sauce, to taste

Directions

- Step 1. Sauté ginger and garlic in sesame, coconut, or olive oil for a few minutes.
- Step 2. Add broth and bring it to a rolling boil. Cook 10–15 minutes to infuse broth with garlic and ginger. While broth is simmering, prepare noodles according to package directions.
- Step 3. Add greens and meat and simmer until cooked, 3–5 minutes. Place noodles in bowls and ladle soup over noodles. Add soy sauce or fish sauce to taste.

Tips and Variations

1. Add any other veggies you want—mushrooms, scallions, string beans, broccoli, carrots, etc.
2. Many Asian soups are spicy. Add some fresh chilies in step 1 or hot sauce like Sriracha in step 3 for some added heat and flavor.
3. Top with bean sprouts, herbs like cilantro, parsley, or mint, and add a squeeze of lemon or lime.
4. If you have an allergy or sensitivity to soy (and if you don't like fish sauce), you can substitute coconut aminos for soy sauce in any of these recipes. Coconut aminos is a soy-free seasoning made from coconut tree sap. You can find good quality products in most health food stores as well as a recommended product on my broths and soups resources page:

http://fearlesseating.net/fearless-broths-and-soups-resources

Thai Coconut Curry Chicken Soup

I don't think it's humanly possible to dislike this recipe. The coconut milk and added sugar make this sweet! Considering this book emphasizes real broths and good-quality ingredients, you might be surprised to see added sugar in this recipe (and the next one). However, sugar is quite common in Asian cuisine, including noodle soups. In the presence of a real broth with other ingredients, sugar is metabolized more slowly than, say, a soda on an empty stomach or a sugary breakfast cereal followed by a sugary coffee drink.

And the problem with sugar isn't sugar itself, but rather *refined* white sugar, which is detrimental to human health when overconsumed. There are now many types of less refined, organic sugars available. In particular, a good match for this recipe would be coconut sugar, which comes from the coconut tree. In Asia, palm trees (which include the coconut tree) are tapped for their sap in the same way that maple trees are tapped in the northeastern United States. The sap is boiled into syrup and then made into sugar. If you can't find coconut sugar, use another type of good-quality organic cane sugar. See my broths and soups resources page for a list of good-quality sugars.

Bottom line, you don't have to fear sugar in small quantities from good sources! This recipe is a great way to enjoy sweetness in a healthy fashion.

Ingredients

- 1 quart chicken broth
- 2 (14-ounce) cans coconut milk
- Cooked chicken of your choice (legs, breasts, thighs), sliced into strips
- 2–3-inch piece of ginger, diced
- About 1–2 Tbsp Thai red curry paste (see Tips and Variations below for sources), less or more for desired flavor and spiciness
- Rice noodles

Accompaniments

- Fish sauce, to taste (I add about 1 Tbsp per bowl)
- Coconut sugar or organic cane sugar, to taste (I add about 1 tsp per bowl)
- Lime wedge
- Fresh cilantro or Thai basil

Directions

- Step 1. Add the chicken broth and ginger to a sauce pan and simmer gently about 10 minutes. Add the coconut milk to the chicken broth and simmer a few minutes more. While broth is simmering, prepare rice noodles according to package directions. Drain and rinse with cool water and set aside.
- Step 2. Remove about ¼ cup of the broth to a separate bowl and mix in the curry paste. Return to sauce pan and thoroughly mix. Taste and add more if you desire more spice.
- Step 3. Add chicken and simmer a few minutes, until cooked through. Place a handful of noodles in bowls and ladle soup over noodles. Season to taste with sugar, fish sauce, and lime. Top with fresh cilantro or Thai basil.

Tips and Variations

1. Add any veggies you want.
2. Adjust the amount of coconut milk to your liking. One 14-ounce can may be enough.
3. Pork, beef, and seafood are all commonly used in different coconut curry recipes in Thai cuisine. They would all work in place of chicken here.
4. Different types of Thai curry pastes are commonly available in American supermarkets. A green or yellow (also called massaman) curry paste would work just as well here in place of the red. Green is often a spicier, and yellow is usually sweetened (so additional sugar may not be necessary). See my broths and soups resources page for a few recommended Thai curry paste products.

http://fearlesseating.net/fearless-broths-and-soups-resources

"Taiwanese" Pork Noodle Soup

This recipe was inspired by a Taiwanese beef noodle soup recipe, and it's a good example of how soup recipes can be easily altered. When I found the original recipe, I wanted to make it as written, but I didn't have half the ingredients. And I didn't want to go to the store to get them. I was hungry and cranky and I wanted it NOW. So I improvised with what I had. The result was something completely different than the original recipe. I have no idea if this recipe is truly Taiwanese or not. My taste buds don't care, and yours won't either, because in the end all that matters is that this noodle soup is *absolutely phenomenal.*

Ingredients

- 2 quarts chicken or pork broth
- ¼ cup rice wine or mirin
- 3–4-pound piece of pork, cooked separately and sliced any way you want
- 2 baby bok choy, chopped
- 2–3-inch piece of ginger, sliced
- 4–6 cloves garlic, diced
- 2 Thai red chilies or chilies de arbol, de-seeded and chopped
- 4–6 whole star anise pods
- 1 tsp whole black peppercorns
- Noodles of choice

Accompaniments

- Cilantro, chopped
- Soy sauce, to taste
- Coconut sugar or organic cane sugar, to taste
- Sriracha (or any hot sauce), to taste

Directions

- Step 1. Combine chicken or pork broth, rice wine, ginger, garlic, chilies, anise, and black pepper in a sauce pan, cover and simmer gently, 30–60 minutes. While broth is simmering, prepare noodles. Add bok choy with the noodles in the boiling water in the last few minutes and simmer a few minutes till tender. Drain and run cool water over noodles and bok choy. Set aside.
- Step 2. Place noodles and bok choy in soup bowls, top with pork, and ladle broth over. Season to taste with accompaniments.

Tips and Variations

1. Sub chicken for the pork for a "Taiwanese" chicken noodle soup!
2. The Thai red chilies in this soup are VERY spicy! The two I use are just enough to give the soup a solidly spicy boost without it being overpowering. But that's just my personal preference. Exclude them if you're not a fan of spicy. Or add more!
3. Because this soup has a spicy kick, I love the addition of a little sugar to complement the spice. I add about a teaspoon per bowl. But you could certainly leave out the sugar entirely. Or add more!
4. Experiment with different herbs and seasonings. Add in a cinnamon stick. Throw in some cloves or fennel seeds. A little of this or that won't ruin your soup. It will only enhance it!
5. Chinese egg noodles work well in this recipe. I often use udon.

Asian Beef Noodle Soup

This recipe involves a slightly more involved take off the basic three-step formula. In particular, step 3 requires the beef to be prepared by a quick searing on both sides.

Ingredients

- 2 quarts beef broth
- 1–1 ½ pound flank steak, cut into strips
- 3–4 tsp sesame oil (http://amzn.to/N8qtts)
- 4–8 cloves garlic, finely chopped
- 3–4-inch piece of ginger, peeled and chopped
- 1 bok choy, chopped (separate and set aside the green leafy ends from the whiter stalks)
- 1 large red pepper, de-seeded and thinly sliced
- 15–20 shiitake mushrooms, sliced
- 1 package noodles of your choice—udon and soba noodles work well
- 3–4 Tbsp soy sauce (http://amzn.to/1fynlyC)

Directions

- Step 1. Sauté garlic and ginger in half the sesame oil for about 5 minutes.
- Step 2. Add beef broth, soy sauce, mushrooms, red pepper, and bok choy stalks to broth and simmer for 5–10 more minutes. Add the bok choy greens in the last minute as they'll cook much quicker than the stalks. While all this is simmering, prepare noodles according to package directions; drain in cold water.
- Step 3. Lightly sear the flank steak in the rest of the sesame oil, 2–3 minutes per side so that the outside is nice and brown but the inside is still pink. It's best to undercook it because it will cook a bit more when you add the hot broth. You can also grill or broil the steak. Remove from heat and slice the steak across the grain,

into strips of any size you prefer. Put several beef strips and a handful of noodles in serving bowls and ladle broth with vegetables over. Add more soy sauce, if needed, to taste.

Tips and Variations

1. Serve with a side of kimchi or add the kimchi right in the soup.
2. Add some hot chilies or hot sauce for extra heat.
3. Other cuts of beef will work fine. I've used strip steak, sirloin, and even leftover pieces from a roast.
4. Many Asian recipes call for thin strips of beef in soups. I find they tend to overcook when the hot broth is added. For this reason, I tend to slice the steak into slightly thicker strips, about a ¼-inch thick.
5. Shiitake mushrooms are great here, but they're a little pricier than most mushrooms. Feel free to use any type of mushrooms in their place.

Chicken Udon Noodle Soup

Besides ginger and garlic, there's another magical combination that tends to work beautifully in Asian noodle soups—cinnamon and whole star anise. You'll see them in many noodle soup recipes, and I consider them the shining star in this one. Ideally, you want to use a cinnamon stick. You could also use cinnamon powder, but just know that it will cloud the soup a bit. No big deal in my book (literally speaking).

Ingredients

- 2 quarts chicken broth
- 2 Tbsp rice wine or mirin, optional
- Any type of chicken you prefer (legs, thighs, breasts, etc.), shredded, sliced, or chopped
- 1 Tbsp lard, sesame, olive or coconut oil
- 3–6 cloves garlic, diced
- 2–4-inch piece of ginger, diced
- 4 ounces mushrooms of your choice
- ¼ head napa cabbage, cut into strips
- 3–4 whole star anise pods
- 1 cinnamon stick
- 1 package noodles of your choice (I prefer udon in this one)
- Soy sauce, to taste
- Sriracha or other hot sauce, to taste

Directions

- Step 1. Sauté garlic, ginger, and mushrooms in oil for about 5 minutes.
- Step 2. Add chicken broth, rice wine, star anise, and cinnamon stick and simmer for 10–15 minutes. While broth is simmering, prepare noodles according to package directions.
- Step 3. Add chicken and cabbage and simmer a few minutes, until cabbage is wilted and tender and chicken is cooked through. Ladle into bowls and season to taste with soy sauce and/or hot sauce.

Tips and Variations

1. As much as I love star anise and cinnamon here, it's OK to skip them. The base of ginger, garlic, broth, and soy sauce will more than make up for it.
2. No big whoop if you don't have the rice wine. It does add a nice subtle flavor, though.
3. Substitute Chinese five-spice powder for star anise and cinnamon. Five-spice powder is a common spice mixture in Asian cuisine that consists of star anise, cinnamon, cloves, fennel seeds, and Sichuan pepper. You'll find it in the spices section of many larger health food stores like Whole Foods and always in Asian supermarkets. Use about 1 Tbsp in this recipe.
4. Add poached, hard-boiled, or soft-boiled eggs in place of or in addition to the chicken.
5. Possible garnishes: fresh chilies, cilantro, scallions, parsley, lemon.

Ginger-Miso-Sesame Soup with Soba Noodles

This is a great example of a miso soup that's not a typical light miso soup. Choose whatever type of miso paste you prefer and add as much or as little as you want. Start slowly, add just a little paste, and taste the soup. Continue to add more paste in small increments if needed for more flavor but know that this soup has many other elements that will complement the miso. I really love soba noodles here. You could use other noodles for sure but the nutty flavor of soba pairs well with the sesame oil.

Ingredients

- 2 quarts chicken broth
- 3–4 tsp sesame oil
- 2–3-inch piece of ginger, diced
- 2–4 cloves garlic
- 2–3 scallions, chopped, bottom white part and leafy green part separated
- 4–8 ounces mushrooms of your choice
- Greens of your choice
- 1 package soba noodles
- 1–2 Tbsp miso, less or more to taste
- Soy sauce, to taste, optional

Directions

- Step 1. Sauté ginger, garlic, white part of scallions, and mushrooms in half of the sesame oil, about 5 minutes.
- Step 2. Add broth and simmer 5–10 minutes. Remove about ½ cup, dissolve in miso, add back to soup, and mix well. Taste and add more miso in the same manner, if needed. While broth is simmering, prepare noodles. Drain and rinse in cool water and set aside.
- Step 3. Add greens and chopped green part of scallions and simmer a few minutes. Place noodles in bowls and mix with the rest of the sesame oil, adding more or less

according to taste. Pour broth over and season to taste with soy sauce.

Tips and Variations

1. A little note about the use of sesame oil: sesame oil is about as common in Asian cuisine as olive oil is in Mediterranean cuisine. Its nutty flavor is a perfect complement to many Asian dishes. But it's commonly shunned as a cooking oil in nutrition circles because it's high in omega-6s, a type of essential fatty acid that doesn't stand up well to heat and oxygen. However, *cold-pressed, unrefined* sesame oil has naturally occurring antioxidants that keep it relatively stable, and thus it is fine to use for light heating applications like stir frying. *Toasted* sesame oil, which is darker in color and enhances the nutty flavor, is not as heat stable and is best to use more as a seasoning.
2. Add chicken or hard-boiled or soft-boiled eggs for a protein boost.
3. Sub fish broth and add any seafood you want. Shrimp, in particular, works well.
4. Add any veggies you want. Red or yellow pepper will add nice color if you're into making things look pretty. Needless to say, I am not.

Faux Pho

Pho (pronounced "fuh") is sort of like the mohinga of Vietnam. It's widely popular throughout the country, is commonly served as breakfast, and has tons of regional variations. But at its core, pho is basically three things. The first is an incredibly fragrant beef broth infused with some aromatic spices and charred onions and ginger. Second, the broth is poured over beef and rice noodles. And third, it's topped with a variety of garnishes including Sriracha sauce, hoisin sauce, fish sauce, bean sprouts, lime, and herbs like cilantro and Thai basil.

Traditional versions call for the spices to be toasted and the onions and ginger to be charred. They're then added to the broth and simmered for 4–10 hours. For a quicker version, my faux pho skips roasting the onion and ginger, toasting the spices, and simmering them for hours on end in the beef broth. Instead, I add the spices and some sliced ginger to the broth and simmer everything for about 30–60 minutes. Though this broth certainly won't take on the complexity of flavor of a more traditional one, it's a *thousand times better* than anything you can buy in a box or a can. Also, because I don't consume this all at once, the broth will develop more flavor as the ginger and spices remain in the broth. This is why I don't remove them after the shorter simmering time.

Finally, you can more than make up for a perfectly fragrant broth with the garnishes. For me, that's where the magic really happens. A little fish sauce, a little Sriracha and hoisin sauce, a squeeze of lime, a handful of bean sprouts, and some fresh herbs really bring things to life

As far as I'm concerned, this faux pho version is not too distant from the more traditional version. Purists would surely disagree, but I'm not interested in being a purist. I'm interested in quick, simple, and delicious. This faux pho recipe fulfills all three.

Ingredients

- 2 quarts beef broth
- Flank steak, London broil, or sirloin steak, sliced as thinly as possible across the grain
- Rice noodles

Spices

- 2–3-inch piece of ginger, diced
- 1–2 cinnamon sticks
- 4–6 whole star anise pods
- 4–6 whole cloves
- 4–6 whole cardamom pods
- 1 tsp fennel seeds
- 1 tsp coriander seeds

Accompaniments

- Fish sauce, to taste
- Sriracha, to taste
- Hoisin sauce, to taste
- Handful each fresh mint, basil, and/or cilantro
- Handful bean sprouts
- 1 lime wedge

Directions

- Step 1. Put spices in a small mesh bag, tea bag, or any thin piece of cloth that you can tie up and secure the spices inside. Alternatively, you can just add them loosely to the broth and strain them out later. Simmer beef broth with ginger and spices for 30–60 minutes. Keep lid on pot, otherwise the stock will evaporate. While broth is simmering, prepare rice noodles according to package directions and set aside.

- Step 2. Put rice noodles and thin beef strips in bowl. Pour hot broth over them. The heat will cook the beef. Add accompaniments to taste.

Tips and Variations

1. You could certainly make a more traditional broth for pho by adding in all the spices and the ginger when you make your beef broth from scratch. Just know that your entire broth will now be a broth for pho. That could be A LOT of pho. Go pho it if you want.

2. Traditionally, pho often includes several different cuts of meat including flank steak, brisket, and tendons and meat from the bones. Some of these are cooked in the broth and some are served raw on the side. I forego the cooked pieces and mostly use raw flank steak to keep things simple. You could also use other cuts like London broil or strip. Whatever you use, slice it super thin, across the grain, so that it cooks quickly in the hot broth.

3. Broth for pho is best not too heavy and gelatinous. You can thin out a more gelatinous broth for pho with water.

4. I love mint in pho. Cilantro and Thai basil are more commonly used herbs. Use whatever you want. Or combine all three!

5. If you have time, go ahead and char some onions and ginger and throw them in with the broth. It will definitely add a wonderful smoky flavor.

6. Be sure to check out my broth and soups resources page for my favorite brand of fish sauce, which is made in the traditional method in Vietnam. Most fish sauce brands are highly processed with added chemicals and MSG.

Asian Pork Chop Noodle Soup

I love using pork chops in noodle soups because unlike other cuts of pork, in the same time it takes the broth to simmer, the pork chops can be broiled quickly on each side, sliced into strips, and ready to go. Udon noodles go really well in this soup!

Ingredients

- 2 quarts chicken or pork broth
- 2 pork chops, broiled and cut into strips
- 2–4 Tbsp soy sauce
- 3–4 Tbsp fat of your choice—lard, butter, sesame, or olive oil
- 2 carrots, chopped
- 1 medium white onion, chopped
- 2–3-inch piece of ginger, peeled and chopped
- 3–6 cloves garlic, chopped
- ½ pound shiitake mushrooms or mushrooms of your choice, chopped
- ½ head Chinese cabbage, chopped into strips
- Udon noodles

Accompaniments

- 1 bunch cilantro, chopped
- Lemon or lime wedges
- Soy sauce
- Sriracha or other hot sauce, optional

Directions

- Step 1. Heat fat in a stockpot over medium heat and add carrots and onion until softened and slightly browned. Add the garlic and ginger and sauté a few more minutes. Add the mushrooms and cabbage and sauté a few more minutes. Add more fat if necessary.
- Step 2. Add the broth and soy sauce, cover, and simmer gently about 15–20 minutes. While broth is simmering, prepare both the noodles (according to package directions) and pork chops. Coat pork chops with olive oil and season with salt and pepper. Broil about 5–6 minutes per side until cooked through. Set aside and let cool. Slice the pork chops into strips.
- Step 3. Place a handful of noodles in bowls and ladle soup over noodles. Add the pork on top. Add accompaniments to taste.

Burmese Coconut Chicken Noodle Soup

I stumbled across this noodle soup only a few times in Yangon, but it left a lasting impression. It has many similarities to mohinga, one of them being the use of chickpea flour (also called fava) as a mild thickener. Combined with the coconut milk and chicken broth, it gives this soup a deeply satisfying, earthy sweetness.

Ingredients

- 1 quart chicken broth
- 2 (14-ounce) cans coconut milk
- Chicken of your choice (legs, breasts, thighs), sliced into strips
- 1–2 Tbsp coconut oil
- 1 large red onion, sliced
- 4–6 cloves garlic, minced
- 3–4-inch piece of ginger, minced
- 2–3 tsp turmeric
- 1–2 tsp paprika
- ¼ cup chickpea flour, a little less or more to desired consistency
- 1 package noodles of choice
- Salt, to taste

Optional Accompaniments

- Hard-boiled or soft-boiled eggs
- 1 avocado, sliced
- Fresh cilantro, chopped
- Lemon or lime wedges
- Pinch or two of roasted chili powder
- Sriracha sauce

Directions

- Step 1. Sauté onion in coconut oil about 5–7 minutes, until browned but not charred. Add garlic and ginger and sauté another 5 minutes, stirring frequently. Be careful not to burn them. Next, add turmeric and paprika, mix and sauté another minute or two.
- Step 2. Add chicken broth and bring to a simmer. Ladle out a few cups of the broth into a separate bowl, add the chickpea flour, and mix well. Drizzle the mixture into the soup, stirring to prevent clumps. Simmer another 5–10 minutes. Taste and add more turmeric or paprika if needed. While broth is simmering, prepare noodles according to package directions.
- Step 3. Add coconut milk to soup and stir. Add chicken and simmer a few minutes. Place noodles in soup bowls and ladle soup over noodles. Season to taste with salt. Add accompaniments to taste.

Tips and Variations

1. Personally, I love all of the accompaniments, but the one I would HIGHLY recommend is some avocado slices as they're a perfect complement to this soup. I'm not a fan of importing fruit (yes, avocado is a fruit!) from halfway around the world, but I wouldn't object to someday having Burmese avocados in our supermarkets. The size of softballs, you'll never be able to look at a wimpy Hass avocado the same way ever again.
2. Use eggs in place of chicken for a Burmese coconut curry egg noodle soup! Do the same with beef and beef broth.
3. Leave out meat and eggs entirely. This will still be very filling!
4. Eggs noodles work best in my opinion, though I've used both udon and rice noodles.

Want more Asian noodle soup recipes?

Download them for free here:

http://www.fearlesseating.net/fearless-broths-and-soups-bonus-recipes

Chapter 20

Simple Sausage and Meatball Soups

In this chapter, I focus on soups that use ground meat, in particular, sausage and meatballs, which are staples in traditional soups all over the world. Ground meats are without a doubt the most affordable cut of meat, and good-quality ground meats from grass-fed and pastured animals are not much more expensive than conventional sources. They're also a great way to get a super hearty soup on the table REALLY FAST. Affordable, nourishing, and fast? *That's* what this book is all about.

Sausages in particular are the easiest type of ground meat to use. Some come precooked like kielbasa or linguica. All you have to do is chop them into rounds, add them to a simmering soup, and they're ready in less than a minute. Others are freshly prepared. If you're short on time, you can also chop them up, add them to the simmering broth, and they'll cook in just a few minutes. If you have more time, browning them in some oil or even roasting or grilling them will create a deeper flavor. Experiment with any types of sausage you want in these recipes. Most stores will offer a wide variety with different spices and seasonings. Though pork is the most common type of ground meat in sausage, you'll also find varieties with ground chicken, turkey, and beef. Use whatever you want!

Meatballs take a little more time to prepare, but it is well worth preparing a large batch at once. I often use two pounds of ground meat and prepare as many meatballs as I can from that. That makes A LOT of meatballs. Whatever I won't use immediately goes in the fridge for the coming week. All I have to do is warm up the leftover soup, throw in some fresh meatballs, simmer them a few minutes, and it's ready in five minutes. At two quarts of broth per pot of soup, I often get an additional five to six five-minute meals throughout the week.

Portuguese Kale Soup

Hands down, this is the soup I make most frequently with sausage. Traditionally, it uses either chorizo (also called chourico) or linguica sausage. Chorizo sausage is spiced with dried hot red pepper and will infuse the broth with a red color and a rich, smoky, and spicy flavor. Linguica is smoke-cured (and thus precooked) and only mildly spicy. Substitute any sausage you want if you're not a fan of spiciness.

Ingredients

- 2 quarts beef broth
- 3–4 links chorizo or linguica sausage, chopped into rounds
- 1–2 Tbsp butter, lard, or tallow
- 3–4 cloves garlic, diced
- 1 onion, diced
- 3–4 carrots, peeled and diced
- 3–4 stalks celery, diced
- 1 bunch kale, chopped
- 1–2 Tbsp dried oregano
- 2 bay leaves
- Salt and pepper, to taste

Directions

- Step 1. Sauté garlic, onion, carrots, and celery in butter, lard, or tallow for 10–15 minutes over medium heat.
- Step 2. Add beef broth, oregano, and bay leaves, bring to a boil, reduce heat, and simmer 10–15 minutes.
- Step 3. Add sausage and kale, simmer 5–7 minutes, until sausage is cooked through and kale is wilted and cooked down. Season to taste with salt and pepper.

Tips and Variations

1. Put all the ingredients in a slow cooker except the kale and sausage and cook on low for 6–10 hours. When it's ready, sauté the kale and sausage separately, dice and add to the soup.
2. Many Portuguese kale soup recipes included tomatoes, potatoes, and/or kidney beans. Add just one or all of them together.

Italian Meatball Soup

As someone with an Italian mother and two Italian grandmothers, I grew up eating all types of Italian food. I can honestly say that this is one of the best Italian meals I've ever had. Whether you're Italian or not, I'm confident you'll agree.

Ingredients

For the meatballs:

- 1 pound ground beef
- ¼–½ cup grated Parmesan cheese, optional
- 1 egg
- 1 cup bread crumbs, optional
- 2 Tbsp fresh parsley, minced
- 1 tsp dried oregano
- ½ tsp salt
- ½ tsp black pepper
- 2–3 Tbsp olive oil

For the soup:

2 quarts beef or chicken broth
2–3 Tbsp tomato paste
1 onion, diced
2 bay leaves
2–3 sprigs fresh thyme
½ tsp black peppercorns

Accompaniments

- Parmesan cheese, grated
- Fresh parsley, chopped
- Salt and pepper, to taste

Directions

- Step 1. Combine all the ingredients for the meatballs (except the olive oil) in a bowl, mix well, and form into balls with your hands. I'd recommend smaller, bite-sized meatballs. Heat olive oil in a soup pot and brown the meatballs on all sides. After a few minutes, add onions (for the soup) and sauté a few minutes, until softened. Remove meatballs and set aside.
- Step 2. To the onions, add broth, tomato paste, bay leaves, thyme, and peppercorns and bring to a boil. Reduce heat and simmer for about 5–10 minutes.
- Step 3. Add meatballs and simmer a few more minutes, until cooked through. Season to taste with salt and pepper. Ladle into bowls and top with parsley and Parmesan cheese.

Tips and Variations

1. Add some chopped carrots and celery with the onions. Personally, I prefer just onions in this recipe.
2. Add some chopped potatoes in step 2 for some additional starch and heartiness.
3. Add in greens in step 3 such as chard, kale, or spinach.

Lamb Curry Meatball Soup

This recipe uses curry powder, which is a blend of dried spices that commonly includes turmeric, cumin, coriander, fenugreek, and chili peppers. It is commonly used in Indian cuisine and, generally speaking, it is milder than curries found in Southeast Asia. However, there are tons of different types of dried curry blends that exist throughout Asia and beyond. The yellow curry powder found in American supermarkets is not exactly a traditional Indian version, but it's more than adequate to use here. By all means, if you can find different types of curry blends in ethnic markets, try them out! And if you're not a fan of lamb, just substitute ground beef in this recipe.

Ingredients

For the meatballs:

- 1 pound ground lamb
- 2 Tbsp chopped fresh parsley
- 1 tsp dried oregano
- 1 tsp cumin
- 1–2 tsp curry powder
- 1–2 tsp garlic powder
- Generous pinch or two of salt and pepper
- 2–3 Tbsp coconut oil or olive oil

For the soup:

- 2 quarts beef or lamb broth
- 2–3 Tbsp butter or coconut oil
- 2 medium white onions, chopped fine
- 3–4 cloves garlic, minced
- 2 tsp curry powder
- 1 tsp cumin
- 1 tsp paprika
- Pinch cayenne

- 1 bunch kale, chopped
- Salt and pepper
- Parsley, chopped

Directions

- Step 1. Combine all the ingredients for the meatballs (except the coconut oil) in a bowl, mix well, and form into balls with your hands. Heat coconut oil in a sauté pan and brown the meatballs on all sides. Set aside.
- Step 2. Heat butter or olive oil in a stockpot over medium heat, add onions and garlic, and sauté a few minutes, until softened and fragrant. Next, add soup spices and continue to sauté a few more minutes.
- Step 3. Add the broth and simmer a few minutes more. Add the kale and meatballs and simmer about 5 more minutes. Season with salt and pepper to taste. Top with chopped parsley.

Tips and Variations

1. Use ground beef instead of ground lamb for a beef curry meatball soup.
2. Substitute any greens you want for the kale. Or just leave the greens out entirely.
3. Garam masala is a type of Indian spice blend that could be used as a substitute for the more common yellow curry powder. A few other Indian curry blends you might find are Muchi curry powder, Vindaloo curry, and Balti curry.

French Onion Soup with Mini Meatballs

Caramelized onions slowly simmered in broth and topped with melted cheese. It's a wonder that something so simple could be so deeply satisfying. But that's the beauty of French onion soup. Most commonly served as an appetizer, this recipe is easily transformed into a hearty meal with the addition of mini meatballs.

Ingredients

For the meatballs:

- 1 pound ground beef
- 2 Tbsp chopped fresh parsley
- 1 tsp sea salt
- ½ tsp black pepper
- 1 cup bread crumbs, optional
- 1 egg
- 2–3 Tbsp olive oil

For the soup:

- 2 quarts beef broth
- 2–3 Tbsp butter
- 2–3 red or yellow onions, sliced thin
- A few sprigs fresh thyme
- 1 tsp whole black peppercorns
- Sourdough bread slices, optional
- Gruyere or Swiss cheese, shredded
- Sea salt, to taste

Directions

- Step 1. Combine all the ingredients for the meatballs (except the olive oil) in a bowl, mix well, and form into mini meatballs with your hands. Heat olive oil in a sauté pan and brown the meatballs on all sides. Alternatively, bake them at 350°F for 10–15 minutes. Set aside.
- Step 2. Melt butter in stockpot over medium-high heat. Stir in onion, reduce the heat to medium-low, cover, and stir often until softened, about 15–20 minutes. If you have time, 30–45 minutes will caramelize the onions even further and bring out more flavor. The more you can brown the onions the better, but be careful not to burn them. Next, add thyme and peppercorns and cook another minute or two.
- Step 3. Stir in beef broth and simmer uncovered for 20–30 minutes or until the broth is reduced by about a quarter. Add meatballs at the end and simmer a few minutes. At this point there are two options depending on how much time you have:

Option 1: Top with shredded cheese and serve with sourdough bread on the side.

Option 2 (highly recommended!): Preheat oven to 350°F. Spoon soup into oven-safe bowls. Lay sourdough bread on top of soup. Layer cheese on top of bread. Bake in oven for 10–15 minutes, until cheese is melted and slightly browned.

Tips and Variations

1. Substitute chicken broth for beef broth.
2. Many French onion soups include a little dry red wine or white wine. Add about a cup with the broth.

Mexican Meatball Soup

If you like tacos, you'll like this Americanized version of Mexican meatball soup. Simply add your favorite salsa to the broth and blend it together. You'll have an instantly flavored, spicy tomato-based broth. Use a mild salsa if you don't like spicy. Prepare and add the meatballs and then add the accompaniments just as you would in tacos!

Ingredients

For the meatballs:

- 1 pound ground beef
- 1 cup bread crumbs, optional
- 1 egg
- 1 large red onion or 2 medium red onions, minced
- 2–3 cloves garlic, minced
- ¼ cup fresh cilantro, chopped fine
- ½–1 tsp salt
- 1–2 tsp cumin
- Generous pinch chili powder, optional
- 2–3 Tbsp olive oil

For the soup

- 2 quarts beef broth
- 1–2 cups of your favorite salsa
- 3–4 Tbsp tomato paste, for an extra tomato kick, optional
- Salt and pepper, to taste

Accompaniments

- Lime wedges
- Cilantro, chopped
- Avocado, sliced
- Dollop sour cream (see note below)
- Cheddar cheese, shredded
- Tortilla chips, crushed

Directions

- Step 1. Combine all the ingredients for the meatballs (except the olive oil) in a bowl, mix well, and form into balls with your hands. If time allows, heat olive oil in a sauté pan and brown the meatballs on all sides and set aside. If not, just plop them into the soup later.
- Step 2. Combine salsa and broth in a blender and puree until smooth. Return to pan and bring to a simmer. Add tomato paste, if using.
- Step 3. Add meatballs and simmer until cooked through. Ladle into bowls, salt and pepper to taste, and top with your preferred accompaniments.

Tips and Variations

1. Use whatever accompaniments you want in whatever combination. The first time I made this, I ruined it by adding too much lime and sour cream. It made it WAY too sour. The next time I added just a little lime and no sour cream at all. For me, that was perfect.
2. As usual, avocado is HIGHLY recommended.
3. Tortilla chips will turn mushy if they sit in the soup too long. Put just a few on top to start and add more as you go. They add a nice crunch!

Pesto Soup with Sausage and Sundried Tomatoes

WARNING: This soup may cause violence. It is *so good* that you WILL find yourself inhaling multiple bowls like some sort of strung-out drug addict. Temporary nirvana will soak through you. If you do have this with others, know that all conversation will stop. Suspicious glances will shoot around the table and primal thoughts of hoarding will arise. Fights may break out if there's not enough for seconds and even thirds. You have been warned.

Ingredients

- 2 quarts chicken, beef, or pork broth
- 2–3 links mild Italian sausage, whole
- 1–2 Tbsp lard, butter, or olive oil
- 3–6 cloves garlic, diced
- 1 large onion or 2 medium onions, diced
- 1–2 cups sundried tomatoes
- ¼–½ cup pesto
- Parmesan cheese, shredded, optional

Directions

- Step 1. Brown sausage on all sides in butter, lard, or olive oil, about 5 minutes. Add onion and garlic around sausage and sauté a few more minutes. Remove sausage, set aside, and cut into circles when slightly cooled.
- Step 2. Add sundried tomatoes with garlic and onions and cook another minute or two.
- Step 3. Add broth and simmer a few minutes. Next, add in half the pesto, dissolve, and stir. Add more pesto as needed. (I usually add A LOT!) Add in sausage. Ladle into bowls and top with optional Parmesan cheese.

Tips and Variations

1. Pesto is widely available in prepared form, but you could certainly make it yourself. It adds an extra step of course, but it's very easy. I love making pesto at the height of basil season in the late summer and early fall. For a cup of pesto, in a food processor add a few cups of packed basil, 3–4 cloves garlic, ½ teaspoon salt, and ¼ cup of pine nuts or walnuts (walnuts are a lot cheaper). Blend this all together and then, with the blender running, drizzle in about a ½–¾ cup olive oil.

2. Add any short-cut pasta of your choice—macaroni, spiral, penne, orecchiette, etc.

3. Season to taste with salt and pepper, if needed. I find there's little need for this as the pesto usually includes it.

4. Use any type of sausage you want. I like a milder sausage here as to not overwhelm the pesto and sundried tomato flavor.

Sausage and Greens in a Garlic-Ginger Broth with Kimchi

Kimchi is a traditional Korean spicy fermented vegetable dish and is widely available in health food stores. It's often served on the side as an accompaniment, but I love adding it right in Asian-themed soups as it infuses the broth with additional spice and flavors. You could certainly leave it, though, and just have it as a side dish.

Ingredients

- 2 quarts beef broth or chicken broth
- 2–3 Tbsp mirin or Chinese rice cooking wine, optional
- 2 links hot sausage—hot Italian, chorizo, etc.
- 3–6 cloves garlic, chopped
- 2–3-inch piece of ginger, diced
- Greens of choice—kale, spinach, chard, etc.
- Soy sauce, to taste

Optional Accompaniments

- Kimchi
- Hot sauce
- Sesame oil

Directions

- Step 1. Add ginger, garlic, broth, and optional mirin or Chinese rice cooking wine to pot and bring to a simmer for 5–10 minutes.
- Step 2. Add greens and sausage and simmer until sausage is cooked, a few minutes.
- Step 3. Season to taste with soy sauce. Top with optional accompaniments to taste. Keep kimchi on the side, if preferred. I love mixing it right in.

Tips and Variations

1. Add some rice or potatoes to make it more filling.
2. Use a milder sausage if you're not a fan of spice.
3. Sub meatballs for the sausage. Pork meatballs, in particular, would work well.

Sausage Minestrone

Legumes, such as beans and lentils, are commonly included in soups with sausage. But I've chosen to forego the use of them in these recipes for one big reason. Legumes need to be soaked, often for lengthy periods, and then simmered for many hours to make them more digestible. Canned beans don't go through this process, and it's the reason I rarely use them. Of course, using canned beans sure is convenient, and I'd be lying if I didn't say I don't use them on occasion. Minestrone is a classic Italian soup that is so simple to make that this is where I make an exception. Even without the sausage, it's incredibly filling, and you could certainly leave out the sausage if you want.

Ingredients

- 2 quarts beef broth
- 2 links sausage of your choice
- 1–2 Tbsp lard, butter, or olive oil
- 3–4 cloves garlic, diced
- 2 carrots, chopped
- 2 stalks celery, chopped
- 1 (14.5-ounce) can diced tomatoes, preferably with Italian herbs
- 2 (15-ounce) cans kidney beans
- Greens of choice
- Short-cut pasta of choice, optional—macaroni, spiral, penne, orecchiette, etc.
- Parmesan cheese, optional
- Salt and pepper, to taste

Directions

- Step 1. Brown sausage on all sides in lard, butter, or olive oil for about 5 minutes. Add garlic, carrot, and celery with sausage and simmer a few more minutes. Remove sausage and set aside. Chop into circles when slightly cooled.
- Step 2. Add broth and tomatoes and simmer until carrots are tender, about 5–10 minutes. While soup is simmering, prepare pasta, if using.
- Step 3. Add sausage, kidney beans, and greens and simmer a few minutes, until sausage is cooked through. Add optional pasta. Top with parsley and optional Parmesan cheese. Salt and pepper to taste.

Polish Sausage and Cabbage Soup

Most of us think of kielbasa as a smoked, precooked sausage, but in Poland, kielbasa could mean any number of types of Polish sausage. In fact, I read once that there are hundreds of types of kielbasa in Poland. I love using the typical kielbasa here, though, not just for its smoky flavor but also because all you have to do it slice it up and add it to the soup.

Ingredients

- 2 quarts beef or pork broth
- Kielbasa, sliced into rounds
- 1 Tbsp lard, butter, or olive oil
- 1 large or 2 medium white onions
- 3–4 cloves garlic, chopped
- ½ medium green cabbage, chopped into strips
- 2–3 cups chopped potatoes of choice
- Salt and pepper

Directions

- Step 1. Sauté onions in lard, butter, or olive oil about 5 minutes. Add garlic and cabbage and cook another 5–10 minutes, until cabbage is softened.
- Step 2. Add broth and potatoes and simmer until potatoes are tender, about 10–15 minutes.
- Step 3. Add kielbasa and simmer a few minutes. Season to taste with salt and pepper.

Tips and Variations

1. This may sound crazy, but there's nothing wrong with substituting hot dogs in this recipe!
2. Top with some sauerkraut.
3. Add a little dollop of sour cream.
4. Serve with a side of sourdough toast and butter.

Want more meaty soup recipes?

Download them for free here:

http://www.fearlesseating.net/fearless-broths-and-soups-bonus-recipes

Chapter 21

Creamy Vegetable Soups

I f I played a word association game with every American and I said the word "soup," I guarantee you the most common response would be "Campbell's." America's favorite soup company has invested millions of dollars to brainwash us into believing their soups are the real thing. You're surely familiar with their TV commercials. They often feature famous athletes and their moms promoting their soups with a carefully crafted image of maternal love and nourishment.

To see how successful they've been, just take a stroll down the soup aisle of your conventional mega-supermarket. You'll see the same two companies dominating the aisle in every supermarket in every state in America—Campbell's and Progresso. Once, I was curious and so I walked into the local Stop 'n Shop where I live, and I counted every type of soup from both companies. I counted ninety-four varieties of Campbell's and seventy varieties of Progresso. That's over 160 soups from just two companies! Combined they accounted for over 95 percent of the soup choices.

A significant portion of these were creamy vegetable soups. Tomato, cream of mushroom, cream of broccoli, cream of potato, and dozens more are among the bestsellers for these companies. These soups sell well because they're familiar to us. Mothers and grandmothers have been making these from scratch for centuries. Before the age of canned soups, creamy vegetable soups were some of the simplest soups to prepare at home. It doesn't get much easier than simmering some vegetables, adding some broth, and pureeing it all together. That is, of course, with the exception of canned soup. But as we've learned, canned soups, *especially* those from Campbell's and Progresso, are full of trans fats, genetically modified ingredients, and all sorts of artificial and, of course, "natural" flavors.

Unlike the previous chapters, in this one I've chosen to stay "inside the box." Most of these recipes will be familiar. If you grew up eating them from cans, that's OK! I did too. But I hope you'll learn to make these soups the way they're intended to be made—from scratch, with your own homemade broths. I know it's a little more time-intensive than opening up a can, but it's well worth it for your health and your family's health! Your grandmother would be very proud.

Two Things about Creamy Veg Soups That Are a Little Different

The first five recipes below use starchy root vegetables, which create an inherent thick creaminess in these soups. But the second five recipes use more fibrous vegetables, and they include a little flour to help thicken them. These are the only recipes in this book that use flour (except one). If you're gluten-free, there are many gluten-free flours on the market that you can use as a substitute. Some work better than others for thickening, but I've found that either a brown rice flour or an all-purpose gluten-free flour work well.

Finally, all of these soups are pureed. I would HIGHLY recommend an immersion blender because you can puree the soup right in the pot. They're very affordable, and you can find them on Amazon or any local kitchen supply store (see my recommended choice on my broths and soups resources page: http://fearlesseating.net/fearless-broths-and-soups-resources). You can also use a regular blender, though it's a bit more time-consuming and often messy. You'll have to transfer batches from your soup pot to the blender and then transfer them back to the soup pot. Be careful when blending a hot soup in a blender! It can easily splatter and burn your skin. Keep the blender cover tightly secured with a thick kitchen towel or oven mitt.

Potato Leek Soup

Potatoes are, without a doubt, the simplest root vegetables to use for creamy vegetable soups. Their starchiness creates a natural creaminess all on its own. Though you can add cream, you don't have to! And if you don't have leeks, any type of onion will work fine.

To make this recipe truly memorable, include the accompaniments. I love fresh chives in the spring and a dollop of sour cream for an extra boost of creaminess. But nothing pairs better than bacon. It adds a salty, smoky flavor that will elevate this from simple goodness to epic greatness. Not even Campbell's and their arsenal of "natural flavors" could come up with a recipe as good as this one.

Ingredients

- 2 quarts chicken broth
- 1–2 Tbsp butter
- 2–3 leeks sliced thin
- 3–4 pounds potatoes of your choice, chopped
- Salt and pepper, to taste
- Herbs of your choice—dill, parsley, thyme, and basil all work well

Optional Accompaniments

- Bacon, cooked separately and chopped into bite-sized pieces
- Crème fraîche or sour cream
- Chives, chopped

Directions

- Step 1. Sauté leeks in butter a few minutes, until soft but not browned.
- Step 2. Add chicken broth and potatoes and bring to a boil. Reduce heat, cover, and simmer about 15–20 minutes, until potatoes are tender. Puree with an immersion blender or handheld blender.
- Step 3. Add herbs and simmer for another 5 minutes. Season to taste with salt and pepper. Serve with optional accompaniments.

Tips and Variations

1. If you don't mind a chunkier version, forget any sort of blender and just mash the potatoes with a potato masher and mix well.
2. Adjust amount of broth for a thinner or thicker consistency.
3. Add heavy cream with the herbs and vegetables in step 3 for additional creaminess. You could also add some coconut milk in place of cream.

Sweet Potato Coconut Curry Soup

I'd just come home from my veggie CSA with more sweet potatoes than I knew what to do with. But after I sampled a butternut squash coconut soup at Whole Foods (gotta love the free samples at Whole Foods), I knew I had my answer. I subbed the sweet potatoes for the squash, threw in some curry to liven it up, and topped it with some crème fraîche for an extra dose of creamy goodness. Boom. A sweet potato coconut curry soup recipe. So very simple and so very hearty and nourishing.

Ingredients

- 1 quart chicken broth
- 1 (14-ounce) can coconut milk
- 1–2 Tbsp coconut oil
- 3–4 pounds sweet potatoes, peeled and cut into large chunks
- 1 medium white onion
- 2–4 cloves garlic
- 2-inch piece of ginger
- 1–2 Tbsp curry powder
- Salt and pepper, to taste

Optional Accompaniments

- Crème fraîche
- Parsley, chopped

Directions

- Step 1. Mince the onion, garlic, and ginger, preferably in a food processor. Heat coconut oil over medium heat and sauté onion, garlic, and ginger about 5–7 minutes, until softened and fragrant. Add curry powder, mix well, and sauté another minute.
- Step 2. Add the chicken broth and sweet potatoes and bring to a boil. Reduce heat, cover, and simmer about 15–20 minutes, until sweet potatoes are tender. Puree with an immersion blender or regular blender, or mash with a potato masher.
- Step 3. Add coconut milk, mix well, and simmer a few more minutes. Add salt and pepper to taste. Ladle into bowls and top with optional accompaniments.

Tips and Variations

1. Add less broth and less coconut milk for a thicker consistency and vice versa.
2. Add less broth and MORE coconut milk for a more coconutty (yes, coconutty) flavor.
3. Add some chili powder or chili flakes for a little more zing.
4. Add more curry powder for more curry flavor and vice versa, or just leave it out entirely if you're not a curry fan.

Butternut Squash Soup with Gorgonzola Cheese and Pears

This recipe comes courtesy of my roommate, Janice. When I asked her if she had any soup recipes that she truly loved, this one was the first one she mentioned. After I tried it, I knew I had to include it. I've made butternut squash soup many times with many different ingredients, but nothing beats the perfect combo of gorgonzola cheese and pears. Serve with a side of toasted sourdough bread and butter for an extra dose of perfection.

Ingredients

- 1 quart chicken broth
- 1 pint heavy cream
- 1 stick butter
- 1 small onion, diced
- 3–4 stalks celery, diced
- 1 butternut squash, halved lengthwise, de-seeded
- 2 Tbsp maple syrup
- Salt and pepper, to taste
- 1 pear, sliced into strips
- Gorgonzola cheese

Directions

- Step 1. Place butternut squash cut side down on baking sheet and bake at 350°F for 45–60 minutes, until tender. Remove and let cool.
- Step 2. Sauté onion and celery in butter for 10–15 minutes. While simmering, separate peel from squash and cut squash into smaller pieces. Add to pot with chicken broth and maple syrup. Simmer another 10–15 minutes. Puree with immersion blender or regular blender.
- Step 3. Add cream and mix well. Ladle into bowls and season with salt and pepper. Top with gorgonzola cheese crumbles and pear slices.

Tips and Variations

1. You could certainly blend the gorgonzola cheese and pears with the rest of the ingredients in step 2.
2. Add some ginger and/or cinnamon.
3. Add fresh herbs like dill or parsley.
4. Add a dollop of crème fraîche in place of gorgonzola cheese.

Creamy Carrot-Apple Soup with Cinnamon

Rich (but not too rich) and sweet (but not too sweet), this soup works any time of the year but is especially suited for autumn when apples are in season. It's also especially well-suited for kids as most will find the sweetness in this recipe very palatable. This recipe could also teach kids a lot about preparing real food at home from real farms. Make a whole day of it! Take them apple picking, pick up some carrots at a farm stand, and make this recipe together as a family.

Ingredients

- 1 quart chicken broth
- 1 cup heavy cream
- 1–2 Tbsp olive oil
- 1 small to medium onion, diced
- 2–4 cloves garlic, diced
- 1–2-inch piece of ginger, diced
- 1–1 ½ pounds carrots, peeled and chopped into 1-inch pieces (about 4–5 cups)
- 1–2 whole apples, peeled, de-seeded, and chopped
- 1 Tbsp cinnamon powder
- Salt and pepper, to taste

Directions

- Step 1. Sauté onions, garlic, and ginger in olive oil until softened, about 5 minutes. Add cinnamon and sauté another minute or two. Add carrots and apples and sauté another few minutes.
- Step 2. Add chicken broth, bring to a boil, reduce heat, and simmer 15–20 minutes, until carrots are cooked. Puree with an immersion blender or regular blender.
- Step 3. Add heavy cream, mix well, and season to taste with salt and pepper. Add more cinnamon if desired.

Tips and Variations

1. Sub curry powder for the cinnamon for a curried carrot-apple soup.
2. Add more or less apples for more or less sweetness.
3. Add more cinnamon if desired.
4. Throw in some herbs like dill, parsley, or sage.

Creamy Beet Soup with Sour Cream and Chives

This recipe could also be called a borscht, but I've never been able to discern the difference between a beet soup and a borscht. As far as I can tell, they're similar, though borscht usually has additional vegetables. I'll give you the option to make either one depending on what you like. If you like sweet, go with just beets. If you want an earthier flavor and a slightly thicker consistency, make it a borscht and include the potatoes and celery. In the end, it doesn't matter what you call it—both versions are fantastic, especially with the sour cream and chives!

Ingredients

- 1 quart chicken broth
- ¼–½ cup heavy cream
- 1 Tbsp olive oil
- 2 large beets or 3–4 medium beets, peeled and chopped
- 2 medium potatoes, optional
- 2–3 stalks celery, optional
- 1 onion, chopped
- 2–4 cloves garlic
- Salt and pepper, to taste
- Sour cream, to taste
- Chives, chopped

Directions

- Step 1. Sauté garlic and onion in olive oil about 5 minutes.
- Step 2. Add chicken broth, beets, and optional potatoes and celery, bring to a boil, reduce heat, and simmer about 40–50 minutes, until beets are tender. Puree with immersion blender or regular blender.
- Step 3. Add heavy cream and mix well. Season to taste with salt and pepper and add sour cream and chives to taste.

Tips and Variations

1. Sub scallions for chives, though there is something particularly perfect about using chives here. Strive for chives!
2. Leave out the heavy cream and simply add in sour cream to your desired creaminess.

Creamy Broccoli-Cheddar Soup

Let's face it, broccoli isn't exactly the most pleasant tasting vegetable. Most kids hate it, and I don't know too many adults that like it either, myself included. Just the thought of eating it on its own makes me cringe. But using it in a soup is a whole different story. Fibrous and cruciferous vegetables, like broccoli, are ideal for soups for two reasons. First, by cooking them, they're a lot easier to digest. And second, by pureeing them with cheese, they can actually taste good! This soup is absolute proof.

Ingredients

- 1 quart chicken broth
- 2 cups heavy cream
- 2 Tbsp butter
- 3–4 heads broccoli, stalks removed
- 1 medium onion, chopped
- 3–4 Tbsp flour
- 8–12 ounces shredded cheddar cheese
- Salt and pepper, to taste

Directions

- Step 1. Sauté onion in butter about 5 minutes, add flour, and whisk for about a minute. Add cream and whisk until smooth.
- Step 2. Add chicken broth and broccoli and simmer until broccoli is tender, about 10–15 minutes. Puree with an immersion blender or regular blender.
- Step 3. Add cheese, mix well, and add salt and pepper to taste.

Tips and Variations

1. Start slowly and stir in the cheese in small amounts until you get your desired cheesiness. I often will use more than 12 ounces! Who doesn't love MORE cheese?
2. Add less broth and a little more flour for a slightly thicker consistency.
3. Top with crispy bacon, chopped into pieces. HIGHLY RECOMMENDED!

Cheddar Corn Chowder

This is the only recipe in this chapter that doesn't have to be blended. You could if you want, but personally, I love chunks of potato and whole corn kernels. Blended or not, corn, potatoes, and cheddar cheese are a match made in creamy soup heaven.

Ingredients

- 1 quart chicken broth
- 1 pint heavy cream
- 1–2 Tbsp butter
- 1–2 pounds potatoes, cubed into small bite-sized pieces
- 1 yellow onion, finely chopped
- 6 ears corn on the cob, cut from the cob OR 2 (15-ounce) cans of corn
- ½ cup flour (¾ cup for a thicker consistency)
- 12–16 ounces shredded cheddar cheese
- Salt and pepper, to taste

Optional Accompaniments

- Bacon, cooked separately and chopped into small pieces
- Parsley, chopped
- Pinch of cayenne pepper

Directions

- Step 1. Heat butter in a stockpot over medium heat. Add onion and sauté until soft, about 5 minutes. Add flour, whisk, and cook about another minute.
- Step 2. Add chicken broth and continue to whisk a few more minutes. Add potatoes. Bring to a boil. Lower heat, cover, and simmer for about 10–15 minutes, until potatoes are tender. Add cream and corn.
- Step 3. Add cheddar cheese, melt, and mix thoroughly. Salt and pepper to taste. Top with optional accompaniments.

Tips and Variations

1. Throw in some diced bell pepper with the veggies.
2. Substitute other cheeses like Monterey Jack, pepper Jack, or Havarti, or make a cheese combo!

Cream of Mushroom with Parmesan

Once you make this recipe and see what a REAL cream of mushroom soup should taste like with *actual natural* mushroom flavor (go figure!), you'll never buy another can of Campbell's cream of mushroom soup ever again. It's just impossible. But that also means that you'll never again use Campbell's cream of mushroom soup as an ingredient in a recipe. Seriously, it is unbelievable (and depressing) just how many recipes use it in things like pasta sauces and chicken dishes. Every time I see this I roll my eyes, shake my head, and let out a big sigh. You'll probably start doing the same thing.

Ingredients

- 1 quart chicken broth
- 2 cups heavy cream
- 2 Tbsp butter or olive oil
- 8–12 ounces mushrooms of your choice, chopped— button, crimini, porcini, shiitake, etc.
- 3–4 shallots, chopped
- 3–4 cloves garlic
- 2–3 Tbsp flour
- 1–2 Tbsp dried tarragon
- Parmesan cheese, grated
- Salt and pepper, to taste

Directions

- Step 1. Sauté mushrooms, shallots, and garlic in butter for about 5–10 minutes, until mushrooms are browned and tender. Add flour, whisk, and cook about another minute.
- Step 2. Add chicken broth, cream, and tarragon and simmer about 5 more minutes. Puree with immersion blender or regular blender.
- Step 3. Top with grated Parmesan and season with salt and pepper.

Tips and Variations

1. Adjust creaminess as desired by adding slightly more or less broth, cream, and/or flour.
2. Use any mushrooms you want or use a blend of different mushrooms!
3. Use thyme or dill in place of tarragon.
4. Skip the Parmesan if need be. However, unless you have a dairy allergy or sensitivity, this would be an egregious offense, one that, in my opinion, should be punishable in a court of law.

Cream of Tomato with Basil

Back to the word association game. While "Campbell's" would probably be the first word most would say in response to the word "soup," the second would probably be "tomato." We've all grown up with Campbell's most popular soup. But once you have your homemade broth prepared, a real homemade tomato soup is just minutes away. And of course, it tastes a million times better. One thing about this recipe is that it does include sugar, which helps balance the acidity of the tomatoes. In fact, Campbell's adds a lot of sugar in their tomato soup. In this recipe, add the sugar slowly, to taste, at the end when you add the salt and pepper.

Ingredients

- 1 quart chicken broth
- ½–1 cup heavy cream
- 2 Tbsp butter
- 2–4 cloves garlic, chopped
- 1 medium onion, chopped
- 4–6 Tbsp tomato paste
- 1 (14.5-ounce) can diced tomatoes
- 2–3 Tbsp flour
- Several sprigs fresh thyme
- 2 bay leaves
- Fresh basil leaves, chopped
- 1–3 Tbsp sugar
- Salt and pepper, to taste

Directions

- Step 1. Sauté garlic and onion in butter about 5 minutes. Add tomato paste and cook another minute or two. Add flour, stir, and cook another minute or two, being careful not to burn.
- Step 2. Add chicken broth, tomatoes, thyme, and bay leaves, bring to a boil, and simmer about 10–15 minutes. Remove thyme sprigs and bay leaves and puree with immersion blender or regular blender.
- Step 3. Add cream, mix well, and season to taste with sugar, salt, and pepper. Top with as many fresh basil leaves as you desire.

Tips and Variations

1. Adjust creaminess as desired by adding slightly more or less broth, cream, and/or flour.
2. Additional accompaniments: sour cream, crème fraîche, bacon, parsley, chives.

Asparagus Chowder

I love asparagus season here in the Northeast. It's the first spring vegetable to appear, and it signals that spring has finally arrived and the worst of winter is finally in the past. But it comes and goes really fast! Only the tender, purplish-green shoots that rise from the ground for a few weeks in April are edible. Once the end is in sight, I'll grab several bunches for the fridge and make it last as long as I can. Enter asparagus chowder. Or as they say here in Massachusetts, "chow-dah"! Asparagus chowder is a great way to use any late season asparagus that's on its last legs and hanging on in your fridge. Asparagus freezes well, so you could always make this recipe later in the year as well.

Ingredients

- 2 quarts chicken broth
- 1–2 pints heavy cream
- 2 Tbsp grass-fed butter (http://amzn.to/1oAVyXC)
- 2 Tbsp extra virgin olive oil (http://amzn.to/1fg0D3L)
- 1 large bunch asparagus or 2 small to medium bunches, tips chopped from stalks and stalks cut into ½-inch pieces
- 2–3 medium potatoes, chopped—russet, Yukon gold, or reds
- 1 whole onion, chopped
- 2–3 cloves garlic, chopped
- ½ cup flour
- Salt and pepper, to taste

Optional Accompaniments

- Bacon, chopped into bite-sized pieces
- Chives, chopped
- Sour cream

Directions

- Step 1. Heat butter and olive oil in stockpot over medium heat. Add onions, garlic, and chopped asparagus stalks to butter and oil and sauté about 5 minutes, until softened. Stir in the flour and cook for another minute.
- Step 2. Add chicken broth and potatoes. Bring to a boil, reduce heat, and simmer until potatoes are soft and soup thickens, about 15–20 minutes. Add asparagus tips and simmer a few more minutes. Puree with immersion blender or regular blender.
- Step 3. Add 1 pint heavy cream and mix well. Add the second pint, if desired, for a creamier version. Salt and pepper to taste. Top with optional bacon, chives, and sour cream.

Tips and Variations

1. If you're using an immersion blender, there may be chunks of asparagus left behind. If you want a smoother consistency, use a regular blender. A Vitamix would be ideal if you have one.
2. Add a few cans of organic corn kernels or frozen bags of corn for an asparagus-corn chowder.
3. Add any meat you want for some extra protein—chicken, shrimp, or sausage work well.
4. You could leave out the flour entirely, though it would be a much thinner consistency. To compensate, you could add a few more potatoes, though this would be more of an asparagus-potato chowder. Nothing wrong with that!

Want more creamy vegetable soup recipes?

Download them for free here:

http://www.fearlesseating.net/fearless-broths-and-soups-bonus-recipes

Chapter 22

Soups from the Sea

This chapter features a wide variety of soups that use fish broth. I've made this a separate chapter because I know most people either love seafood or hate it. If you're in the former category, I know you will love these soups as much as I do. Nothing quite stirs my soul like the taste of the sea in the form of soups made with fish broth. With each succulent slurp, I feel a deep connection to the coastal places I've lived and visited. The recipes here feature some of my favorites from these places, both here in the United States and in Asia. There's a little bit of everything for all the seafood lovers out there.

Now if you're a seafood hater, *please do me a favor*. Please give these recipes a chance! Perhaps you grew up eating icky gross fishy things like frozen fish sticks or, god forbid, Filet-O-Fish sandwiches. The thought of fish broth-based soups may send shockwaves of icky fishiness through you, but I promise these recipes are not full of icky fishiness. Remember, fish broth should not taste fishy but rather bring out subtle hints of fish essence in the broth. Combined with other vegetables, herbs, and spices, soups from the sea feature so many other flavors than just seafood.

In particular, I'd recommend starting with one of the first three recipes. It's hard to dislike a good cioppino, bouillabaisse, or a good ol' fashioned New England clam chowder. They are highly palatable to most Western tastes. After that, the rest of the recipes may not be as familiar, but I'm certain you'll find at least a few that surprise you with how good they taste. In time, you may even find yourself addicted to a few of them. Especially the last one!

Finally, don't forget that fish broth is the cheapest, simplest, and least time-consuming broth to make. And though seafood can be pricey, it doesn't have to be. Many types of fish and shellfish are very affordable, and most of these recipes allow you to choose whatever type of seafood you want to use. As always, make these recipes your own and don't be afraid to experiment and improvise.

Basic Cioppino

Cioppino is an Italian fish stew that combines a variety of seafood in a tomato-based broth. Its straightforward simplicity and variability is what I love about it. Basically, take whatever seafood you want and simmer it in a simple base of fish broth, wine, tomatoes, and herbs. It's really that easy . . . and totally addictive. Throw in a mid-summer oceanside setting, a sunset, good friends and family, and a bottle of wine (or three) for the ultimate cioppino experience. For me, it doesn't get much better than that.

Ingredients

- 1 quart fish broth
- ½–1 cup dry red wine
- ½–1 pound mussels and/or steamer clams
- ½–1 pound shrimp, removed from shells
- ½–1 pound whitefish, chopped into bite-sized pieces
- 2 Tbsp olive oil
- 1 medium white onion, diced
- 3–6 cloves garlic, diced
- 1 (28-ounce) can diced tomatoes
- 4–5 Tbsp tomato paste
- 5–10 sprigs fresh thyme
- 2 bay leaves
- 2–4 Tbsp fresh chopped parsley
- 2–4 Tbsp fresh basil
- Salt and pepper, to taste

Directions

- Step 1. Heat olive oil in a stockpot over medium heat and sauté onion and garlic until softened and fragrant, about 5 minutes.
- Step 2. Add wine, fish broth, tomatoes, tomato paste, and herbs. Bring to a boil, then turn down heat and simmer gently for about 10–15 minutes.
- Step 3. Add the mussels and/or steamers and simmer until the shells open, about 4–5 minutes. Next, add the shrimp and whitefish and simmer until cooked through, about 2–3 minutes. Top with parsley and basil and add salt and pepper to taste.

Tips and Variations

1. Add any seafood you want—lobster, scallops, other types of clams, crab, other types of fish, squid, etc. Cioppino comes from San Francisco, where it was typically eaten with whatever came off the boats that day. Needless to say, the fresher the seafood, the better.
2. Sub a dry white wine for the red wine. Either one will work. I think red goes a little better with the heartiness of this dish, but white wine is commonly used too.
3. For a little kick, throw a teaspoon or two of hot red pepper flakes in with the herbs in step 2.
4. Add some toasted bread on the side for dipping in the broth.

Basic Bouillabaisse

Bouillabaisse (pronounced "boo-ya-base") is a fish stew that originated in France. French versions are often quite fancy and are traditionally served in two courses, one of which includes bread with a garlic mayonnaise known as a "rouille." Of course, we're going to forego all that fancy-schmancy stuff in favor of simplicity. This version is another good example of improvising something a lot more reasonable . . . but no less delicious!

Ingredients

- 2 quarts fish broth
- 1 cup dry white wine
- Seafood of choice, chopped into chunks—shrimp, scallops, crab, clams, mussels, squid, meaty whitefish
- 3–4 Tbsp olive oil
- 1 onion, diced fine
- 1 fennel bulb (also called anise), diced fine
- 3–6 cloves garlic, chopped
- 2–3 ripe tomatoes, chopped
- Herbs of choice—fresh thyme (3–4 sprigs), bay leaves, basil, fennel fronds, ¼ tsp crumbled saffron threads (or a pinch or two of powdered saffron) all work well (see tips below)
- Lemon wedges
- Parsley, chopped
- Salt and pepper, to taste

Directions

- Step 1. Sauté onions and fennel bulb in olive oil about 5–10 minutes. Add garlic and sauté another minute or two.
- Step 2. Add chopped tomatoes, fish broth, wine, and herbs and simmer gently for about 10–15 minutes or until the liquid reduces by about a quarter.
- Step 3. Add seafood and simmer until cooked through. Season to taste with salt and pepper, and top with parsley and a squeeze of fresh lemon wedge or two.

Tips and Variations

1. Although pricey, saffron does add a wonderful color, aroma, and flavor to the broth. Include it if you can. Even better, use fennel fronds (the feathery threads that grow off the fennel bulb) along with the saffron. Paired together with the fish broth, they work *really* well.
2. Instead of a fancy rouille, make some garlic bread. Or just grab whatever type of bread you want and slather on some olive oil or butter.
3. Make this a bouillabaisse pasta by adding any pasta you want. Long-cut pasta like fettucine, spaghetti, and linguini pairs really well.

New England Clam Chowder

The quintessential soup of the northeastern United States, it doesn't get much better than good ol' fashioned New England clam chowder. The basic foundation is so simple—potatoes, bacon, clams, cream, and fish broth or clam juice. From there, variations are prevalent, though as far as I'm concerned, there's one true indicator of a good New England chowder. It has to be *thick and creamy*. Growing up, my favorite clam chowder was from Progresso (I know, ugh), which was really thick and creamy. As I got older and started appreciating more authentic versions, my love of rich and creamy chowder remained. But many prefer a thinner version. If you like it thick, follow my recipe, which uses flour as a thickener and heavy cream. If you like something thinner, exclude the flour or cut the amount in half. You could also use a little more broth or use half and half instead of heavy cream. You can play around with things to get the consistency you want. Regardless, this is a classic because it's so flavorful no matter the consistency.

Ingredients

- 1 quart fish broth
- 3–4 cans chopped clams
- 2 cups heavy cream
- 4–5 Tbsp flour
- 4–6 strips bacon or salt pork
- 1 large yellow onion or 2 medium yellow onions, diced
- 2–3 pounds red potatoes, chopped into bite-sized cubes
- Parsley and/or chives, chopped
- Salt and pepper, to taste

- Step 1. Sauté bacon strips or salt pork for about 5–10 minutes, turning once, until browned (but not burned); set aside and drain on paper towels. Next, add onions to bacon fat and sauté until tender, about 5 more minutes. Add flour and mix well for about a minute.
- Step 2. Add fish broth and stir for a few minutes, until broth thickens. Add potatoes, cover, and simmer until potatoes are tender, about 10–15 minutes. While broth is simmering, chop reserved bacon into pieces.
- Step 3. Add clams and cream to soup and simmer a few minutes more. Top with bacon, parsley, and/or chives and season to taste with salt and pepper.

Tips and Variations

1. For a more authentic version (but a more time-intensive process), boil up some fresh clams (cherrystones, littlenecks, steamers, or quahogs), remove them from their shells, and chop them by hand.
2. You could certainly use clam juice in place of or in addition to the fish broth. Include the juice from the canned clams in step 2 or save the clam juice if you're boiling fresh clams.
3. Add some fresh thyme and a bay leaf or two in step 2.
4. For an extra shot of creamy buttery goodness, melt in a tablespoon or two of butter in step 3.
5. Add in a little Worcestershire sauce and/or hot sauce, to taste.
6. Substitute fish for clams for a fish chowder!

New England-Portuguese Clam Boil Soup

Along the coast of southern Massachusetts there is a huge Portuguese influence, and one of the more common dishes is a fusion dish known as a New England-Portuguese clam boil. It involves boiling some steamer clams, potatoes, and corn along with some hot dogs and Portuguese sausage. It's sort of like the quick version of a more traditional New England clam bake, which is a time-intensive process that involves digging a fire pit on the beach, and though epically memorable, is not something the average Joe is going to whip up for dinner. However, a New England-Portuguese clam boil can be made in about a half hour by anyone, anywhere with just a stockpot and stove top. Though typically not a soup, it easily adapts into one by adding a good dose of fish broth. You may not find fresh local steamer clams in your area, but you can use any combination of seafood that you'd like—other types of clams, mussels, and shrimp all work well.

Ingredients

- 2 quarts fish broth
- 1–2 pounds steamer clams
- 1 package organic hot dogs, sliced into 1-inch pieces
- 2–3 links chorizo or linguica sausage (or other spicy sausage) sausage, sliced into 1-inch pieces
- 3–6 cloves garlic, chopped
- 1–2 pounds potatoes, chopped into cubes
- 1–2 medium yellow onions, diced
- Salt, to taste
- Lemon wedges
- Melted butter on the side for dipping clams, optional

Directions

- Step 1. Rinse clams and then soak in cold water, about 5–10 minutes. Drain, rinse, and soak a few times more to remove sand and dirt.
- Step 2. Add fish broth to stockpot along with garlic, corn, potatoes, and onions and bring to a boil. Turn heat down and simmer until potatoes are almost cooked through.
- Step 3. Add sausage and hot dogs and cook about 5 minutes. Next, add the steamer clams, raise heat, and boil until the shells open, about 5–7 minutes. Discard any clams that don't open. Season to taste with salt and lemon wedges. Serve with optional butter on the side for dipping clams.

Tips and Variations

1. In a typical New England-Portuguese clam boil, fresh ears of corn are boiled with everything else. You could boil a few ears separately here for a nice side dish or cut the corn from the cob and throw the kernels in with the soup in step 2. You could just add some canned corn as well.
2. If you don't want to use the hot sausage, just use the hot dogs and vice versa.
3. Serve with a nice piece of toasted sourdough bread and butter!

Spicy Cilantro-Lime Seafood Soup

When I worked at a seafood restaurant in Homer, Alaska, a young chef made an off-the-cuff Peruvian-inspired seafood pasta for a special one night. It was a slow weeknight, one where the chefs had a little more leeway to experiment. Few customers ordered it, and he never made it again. But it was a hit among the staff, and I'll never forget it. The two things that stood out were the lime and cilantro, which fused beautifully with the creamy sauce swimming with fresh seafood. This recipe is inspired from that memorable creation.

Ingredients

- 1 quart fish broth
- ½–1 pound shrimp, diced
- ½–1 pound mussels
- ½–1 pound whitefish like cod, hake, haddock, or halibut, chopped into bite-sized pieces
- 1–2 Tbsp olive oil or coconut oil
- 1 medium onion, diced
- 2–4 cloves garlic, diced
- 1–2 potatoes, chopped into cubes
- 1–2 medium tomatoes, chopped
- 1 hot pepper (Thai red, jalapeño, serrano, etc.), diced, or 1–2 tsp chili powder, optional
- 1 lime, quartered
- ½ cup cilantro, chopped
- Salt or fish sauce, to taste

Directions

- Step 1. Sauté onion and hot pepper, if using, in olive oil or coconut oil for about 5 minutes. Add garlic and chili powder, if using, and sauté another minute or two.
- Step 2. Add fish broth, tomatoes, and potatoes. Bring to a boil, then reduce heat to a simmer, and cook until potatoes are tender, about 10–15 minutes.
- Step 3. Add seafood, 2 lime wedges, and half of the cilantro and simmer until mussels open, if using, or until seafood is cooked, about 5 minutes. After 5 minutes, remove lime wedges but squeeze the juices into the soup. Season to taste with lime juice from remaining lime wedges and salt or fish sauce. Top with additional cilantro.

Tips and Variations

1. Always play around with different spice levels to find what you like. Personally, I prefer using a chili powder because I can add small amounts and then quickly add more to get my preferred spiciness. Or, if you can't tolerate any spice, just leave it out entirely. Always adjust things to your personal tastes, but don't let your personal tastes keep you from trying new things either!
2. You could use canned tomatoes here, but it will make this more of a tomato-cilantro-lime soup. For that reason, I prefer fresh tomatoes.
3. Use any combination of the shrimp, mussels, and fish you want. Or just use one of them. Add other seafood as well—squid, clams, and different types of fish are perfectly suited as well.

Basic Asian Seafood Soup

This recipe is similar to the basic Asian noodle soup. The only difference is the use of fish broth and whatever seafood your heart desires. Use this basic recipe as a foundation for improvising your own variations with different herbs, seasonings, and spices.

Ingredients

- 2 quarts fish broth
- Any seafood you like—shrimp, scallops, mussels, clam, squid, salmon, whitefish, etc.
- 1–2 Tbsp sesame, coconut, or olive oil
- 2–3-inch piece of ginger, diced
- 3–6 cloves garlic, diced
- Any greens you like
- Soy sauce and/or fish sauce, to taste

Directions

- Step 1. Sauté ginger and garlic in oil until soft.
- Step 2. Add fish stock, bring to rolling boil, and cook 10–15 minutes to infuse broth with garlic and ginger.
- Step 3. Add greens and seafood and simmer until seafood is cooked, a few minutes. Add soy sauce or fish sauce to taste.

Tips and Variations

1. Add other veggies—mushrooms, scallions, napa cabbage, carrots, string beans, etc.
2. Many Asian soups are spicy. Add some chilies or hot sauce like Sriracha for some kick and flavor.
3. Add rice noodles. Cook them separately and then add at the end.
4. Top with bean sprouts, herbs (like cilantro, parsley, or mint), and add a squeeze of lemon or lime.

Thai Coconut Green Curry Seafood Soup

You'll see this soup on almost every menu in every Thai restaurant. In Thailand, there are a kazillion variations depending where you are in the country and what's in season. Play around with the ratio of fish broth to coconut milk. I find a 1:1 ratio is pretty good but sometimes prefer more of a coconut flavor and I'll add less fish broth. Remember, the ingredient amounts in all these recipes can be adjusted to your liking. Sometimes you need to experiment to find what you like. Green curry is very spicy so add only a small amount to start. Adding a little sugar will help balance out the spice.

Ingredients

- 1 quart fish broth
- 2 (15-ounce) cans coconut milk
- 1 pound shrimp, peeled and halved or cut into thirds
- 1 pound whitefish, cut into bite-sized pieces
- 1 Tbsp coconut oil
- 2–3 cloves garlic, chopped
- 2–3-inch piece of ginger, chopped fine
- 1 stalk lemongrass, upper half removed, chopped into 1-inch pieces
- 1 red bell pepper, cut into strips
- 2–3 tsp Thai green curry paste
- 2–3 tsp coconut sugar or organic cane sugar, optional
- Fish sauce or soy sauce, to taste
- Lime wedges
- Cilantro

Directions:

- Step 1. Sauté garlic, ginger, and lemongrass in coconut oil for a few minutes.
- Step 2. Add coconut milk and fish broth, bring to a boil, reduce heat, and simmer about 5 minutes. Remove about ½ cup of liquid and mix in curry paste (start with a small amount, about a teaspoon). Mix back into soup and taste. If more spice is desired, add more curry paste in the same manner. Once you have your desired spiciness, do the same thing with the sugar, adding it in slowly to get your desired sweetness.
- Step 3. Add red pepper, shrimp, and fish and simmer until shrimp and fish are cooked. Season to taste with lime, cilantro, and fish sauce or soy sauce.

Tips and Variations

1. If you're unfamiliar with lemongrass, it's a tropical plant with a lemony scent and flavor that is very common in Southeast Asian cuisine. Don't eat it! It's just added for flavor. Strain out the pieces or just pick them out as you go (which is what I do). Many stores in America now carry it. If you can't find any near you, no big deal. Just sub a little squeeze of lemon at the end.
2. Use any seafood you like with or in place of shrimp and fish.
3. Add in some carrots and mushrooms in step 1.
4. Add in some broccoli florets or string beans with the red peppers. If you like the red peppers more cooked, add them in step 1. I prefer more of a crunch and add them in step 3.
5. Add rice noodles.

Thai Hot and Sour Seafood Soup

This is a very basic version of a Thai staple that also has almost infinite incarnations in Thailand. Basic or not, this soup is so flavorful that the first time I made it, I couldn't contain my excitement. I blurted out, "Yeah, baby!" in total Austin Powers fashion. I added just the right amount of hotness with the chilies, sourness with the lime, and saltiness with the fish sauce. In step 2, you control the final flavor by adding as much citrus and fish sauce as you like. Start slowly and continue adding it in until you've hit the sweet (or should I say, "sour") spot. For me, that's the juice of one lime wedge and at least one teaspoon of fish sauce per bowl.

Ingredients

- 2 quarts fish broth
- 1–2 Tbsp coconut oil
- 2–3 scallions, diced
- 3–4-inch piece of ginger, diced
- 1 large stalk lemongrass, top half removed, bottom half chopped into 1-inch pieces
- 2 Thai red chilies, de-seeded and chopped
- 1–1 ½ pounds shrimp, peeled
- 1 pound fish of choice, chopped into bite-sized pieces
- Lime and/or lemon wedges
- Fish sauce, to taste

Directions

- Step 1. Sauté scallions, ginger, chilies, and lemongrass in coconut oil about 5–10 minutes.
- Step 2. Add fish broth and simmer another 5–10 minutes. Remove lemongrass pieces. Add a generous squeeze of fresh lime and/or lemon and season to taste with fish sauce.
- Step 3. Add shrimp and fish and simmer a few minutes, until cooked through.

Tips and Variations

1. Thai red chilies (also called "bird's eye" chilies) are very small and *very* spicy. They're often one of the hotter chilies you'll find in supermarkets. You can substitute a less spicy type of chili or you can substitute a hot sauce of your liking. Or just leave out the chilies entirely.
2. Throw in some rice noodles to make this a little more filling.
3. Add any seafood you want—squid, mussels, and scallops would work fine.

Korean Gochujang Soup with Seafood

Gochujang (pronounced "go-choo-jong") is a Korean sweet and spicy fermented red pepper paste. Don't let its exotic name intimidate you, because this recipe is really simple! It's also more sweet than spicy, so it's quite palatable even to those who don't like spice. Similar to miso and Thai curry pastes, gochujang is easily dissolved in broth where it quickly infuses it with its characteristic flavor. However, unlike the Thai curry pastes, gochujang is not something you'll find in too many health food stores. You'll either need to find an international/world food market or order some online. See my broths and soups resources page for a few recommended products.

Ingredients

- 2 quarts fish broth
- 1 pound meaty whitefish such as haddock, cod, grouper, pollock, or halibut
- ½ pound shrimp, peeled
- 1 teaspoon sesame oil
- 1–2 teaspoons Korean chili powder or regular chili powder
- 1–2 teaspoons gochujang
- 2–3 cloves garlic, chopped
- 1 bok choy, chopped
- 10–15 shiitake mushrooms or mushrooms of choice
- 2–3 teaspoons fish sauce

Directions

- Step 1. Cut whitefish into cubes and mix thoroughly with chili powder, 1 tsp gochujang, garlic, and sesame oil. Let stand for about 20–30 minutes.
- Step 2. Bring broth to a boil, add fish sauce and vegetables, and simmer for 5–10 minutes.
- Step 3. Add the shrimp and fish and simmer for a few minutes, until cooked through. Taste and add more gochujang paste or fish sauce if additional spice and flavoring is desired. Add bok choy greens or other greens in the last minute of simmering.

Mango-Coconut-Curry Mussels Soup

House guests? Hosting a party? This recipe is what I consider more of a special occasion recipe. It's also well-suited as an appetizer, either in soup form or as more of a mussels dish. Either way, this recipe whips up in just a few minutes, but it's so flavorful that your guests will think you spent hours preparing it. Be sure to wallow in the adoration and praise that will surely come your way. And as with all the recipes here, this recipe is ripe for experimentation. Try more or less coconut milk, fish broth, and mangoes. I like the use of curry powder here, but other curry pastes could be used, or it could work well without curry. This is a fun one. Have a ball with it!

Ingredients

- 1 quart fish broth
- 2 (15-ounce) cans coconut milk
- 3–4 mangoes, peeled and separated from pit
- 2–3-inch piece of ginger, chopped, optional
- 1 pound mussels
- 2–4 teaspoons curry powder
- Lime wedges, on side
- Salt or fish sauce, to taste
- Fresh cilantro, chopped

Directions

- Step 1. Place mangoes, coconut milk, fish broth, and optional ginger in a blender and puree until smooth.
- Step 2. Transfer to stove top, bring to a simmer, and add in curry powder, adding more to taste. Simmer about 5 minutes.
- Step 3. Add in mussels and simmer until shells open. Season to taste with lime, fish sauce or salt, and fresh cilantro.

Tips and Variations

1. Sub Thai red curry paste for curry powder. Or, try it without any curry flavoring. It works quite well even without the spice.
2. Sub shrimp for the mussels. Add in scallops or any fish you want.
3. Experiment with different ratios of coconut milk to fish broth. Maybe leave out the fish broth entirely!
4. Try pineapple instead of mango!

Mohinga!

I couldn't think of a more perfect way to end this book. Now truth be told, I originally had no intention of including a mohinga recipe here. For years, it intimidated me. I knew there was NO WAY I could duplicate the real thing. For starters, I didn't have many of the ingredients. I still haven't found banana stem (which is not the stem of store-bought bananas) anywhere. And I still don't know how the Burmese made those amazing, delicately fried fish cakes. But I decided to get over it and do what I always do—experiment with a simplified version. This recipe was my very first attempt. And I was *thrilled* with the results. It may not be an authentic version, but for the last time, the purpose of this book is not to follow recipes exactly and be "authentic" but rather to experiment and do the best you can with what you've got!

Ingredients

- 2 quarts fish broth
- 1 pound whitefish (catfish is commonly used in Burma)
- 2 Tbsp coconut oil
- 1 large onion or 2 small to medium white onions
- 4–6 garlic cloves
- 3–4-inch piece of ginger
- 1 stalk lemongrass, top half (the thinner, green part) removed, bottom half cut into large chunks
- 2 tsp turmeric
- 1–2 tsp roasted chili powder
- ½ cup chickpea (also called fava) flour
- Rice noodles, cooked according to package directions

Accompaniments

- Fish sauce
- Lime wedge
- Fresh cilantro, chopped

- Fried onions, optional
- Hard-boiled or soft-boiled eggs, optional
- Pinch of chili powder, optional

Directions

- Step 1. Dice onion, garlic, and ginger in a food processor and sauté in coconut oil with lemongrass until fragrant, about 3–5 minutes. Add turmeric and chili powder and sauté another minute.
- Step 2. Add fish broth and bring to a boil. Reduce heat and bring to a simmer. Add chickpea flour and stir until mixed well. Simmer for 10–15 more minutes, until slightly thickened. If using fried onions (which I highly recommend), fry them in coconut oil while soup is simmering. Fry until well browned but not blackened. Drain from oil and set aside.
- Step 3. Add fish and simmer 3–5 minutes, until cooked through. Ladle over rice noodles and season to taste with accompaniments.

Tips and Variations

You know the routine by now. Add more of this, less of that. Exclude this ingredient if you don't have it. Add that ingredient if you want. Be creative. Make it your own. Be a cook, not a chef. Have fun.

Good luck!

Want more soups from the sea recipes?

Download them for free here:

http://www.fearlesseating.net/fearless-broths-and-soups-bonus-recipes

How to Make Bone Broth 101

As a final reminder, if you feel you could use some additional support, be sure to check out my online video course, How to Make Bone Broth 101 at www.HowToMakeBoneBroth101.com.

It includes simple instructional videos for how to make all the broths included in this book. It also includes a private Facebook community forum for asking questions, sharing recipes and tips, and connecting with others (including me!).

And finally. . .

One Small Request

Thanks so much for reading my book! I genuinely hope you found it valuable. If so, I'd greatly appreciate if you could take a moment to write a brief review on Amazon. Reviews mean a great deal to me and will help more people find this book. Campbell's and Progresso aren't going away anytime soon, but if this book helps more people ditch the boxes and cans in favor of REAL broths and soups, then I'll consider that "mission accomplished."

And let's stay connected!

The best way to do that is to subscribe to my e-mail list where I regularly send out free recipes, how-to videos, and health tips. Head on over to my website, www.FearlessEating.net, to subscribe. I also plan on writing more books in the future, and I always notify my subscribers with promotional discounts, giveaways, and freebies. No spam, you have my word!

You can also join me on:

Facebook	facebook.com/FearlessEating
Pinterest	pinterest.com/fearlesseating
Instagram	instagram.com/fearlesseating

In health,

Craig

Get More!

Please visit my website at www.FearlessEating.net and subscribe to my mailing list so that we can keep in touch. I plan to write many books in the future and will notify you of their releases and promotional discounts. No spam, you have my word! You'll also get free recipes, digestive health tips, and more great info to support you on your heartburn-free journey!

About the Author

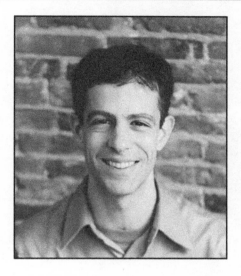

Craig Fear is a certified Nutritional Therapy Practitioner (NTP) who specializes in helping others with chronic digestive issues. He struggled with his own digestive problems for many years, which inspired him to become an NTP and start his practice, Pioneer Valley Nutritional Therapy, in Northampton, Massachusetts, in 2009.

Craig's dietary philosophy is firmly rooted in traditional foods. He believes in real food from small-scale sustainable farms and the pioneering research of Dr. Weston Price as a starting point for what to eat and why.

He also understands dietary changes can be overwhelming for many and has learned to skillfully guide others through the many obstacles modern-day life presents.

He started his blog, Fearless Eating, in 2011 (www.FearlessEating.net), wrote his first book, *The 30 Day Heartburn Solution*, in 2013 (and plans to write many more), and created an online digestive e-course, Fearless Digestion (www.FearlessDigestion.com), in 2014.

Craig's other interests include hiking, playing his guitar, travel, and rooting for his beloved New York Giants. He also loves coffee and claims to be only mildly addicted to it.

Please join Craig over at his blog, Fearless Eating, at www.FearlessEating.net.

CPSIA information can be obtained
at www.ICGtesting.com
Printed in the USA
LVHW090111221219
641378LV00001B/316/P